CANNABIS AND SEXUAL ECSTASY
FOR MEN

"Cliff Dunning's excellent *Cannabis and Sexual Ecstasy for Men* brings exciting news and looks poised to be the go-to guide for men ready to explore what for many of us is untapped potential. The information is well researched and presented in clear, accessible language with just the right amount of layperson-friendly science to frame the instructions. This book promises to be a game changer for any man willing to put the detailed, reliable, and responsibly balanced guidance offered here into practice."

STEPHEN GRAY, EDITOR OF *CANNABIS AND SPIRITUALITY*

"Cliff has done for men what Betty Dodson did for women in her book *Sex for One*—teach you how to master your own orgasm. His well-researched approach will take you step-by-step through using cannabis to heighten your sexual response combined with stimulating the prostate to achieve multiple orgasms. This is definitely a must-read for all men."

NICK KARRAS, PRACTICING SEXOLOGIST
AND AUTHOR OF *THE PASSIONATE HIGH*

"Even without a prostate or natural affinity for cannabis, you'll easily relate to and truly enjoy Cliff's open, honest account of his personal journey to psychoactive sexual awakening, and if you do have either or both, this book might very well be a revelation."

MAMAKIND, CANNABIS COLUMNIST, SEXPERT, AND AUTHOR OF
SEX POT: THE MARIJUANA LOVER'S GUIDE TO GETTIN' IT ON

"Cannabis has an extensive cross-cultural history as an aphrodisiac, notably for increasing sensual awareness. *Cannabis and Sexual Ecstasy for Men* is an essential read on a growing list of books about arousal cultivars (cannabis strains) designed to enhance sexual pleasure and the likelihood of orgasm. This book is a must-read for those interested in new levels of multiorgasmic sexual gratification."

CHRIS BENNETT, AUTHOR OF
CANNABIS AND THE SOMA SOLUTION

"Finally we're speaking openly about this pot-provoked erogenous phenomenon that many of us have been exploring for years. Marijuana does stimulate sexual arousal, and Cliff's book lays bare the many dimensions of cannabis orgasm. The great sexual pioneer Wilhelm Reich insisted that regular orgasms throughout one's life are vital for sustaining emotional and physical health and fulfillment. *Cannabis and Sexual Ecstasy for Men* carries on this essential revolution, nurturing an integration of sexual expression and overall spiritual and psychological well-being."

JOHN SELBY, AUTHOR OF
CANNABIS FOR COUPLES

"I thought I knew pretty much everything about sex and cannabis. I was wrong. The information in this well-written and researched book opens a whole new fascinating chapter on sexual exploration for men and goes a long way toward eliminating the idiotic shame that has been projected onto sexuality and cannabis both."

WILL JOHNSON, AUTHOR OF *CANNABIS IN SPIRITUAL PRACTICE*
AND *BREATHING THROUGH THE WHOLE BODY*

CANNABIS AND SEXUAL ECSTASY
FOR MEN

Awaken the Prostate
for Multiple Orgasms

CLIFF DUNNING

Destiny Books
Rochester, Vermont

Destiny Books
One Park Street
Rochester, Vermont 05767
www.DestinyBooks.com

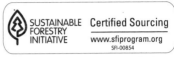

Text stock is SFI certified

Destiny Books is a division of Inner Traditions International

*Note to the reader: This book is intended as an informational guide. The
remedies, approaches, and techniques described herein are meant to supplement,
and not to be a substitute for, professional medical care or treatment. They should
not be used to treat a serious ailment without prior consultation with a qualified
health care professional.*

*The publisher and author are not responsible for any specific health needs that
may require medical supervision and are not liable for any damages or negative
consequences from any treatment, action, application, or preparation to any person
reading or following the information in this book.*

Cataloging-in-Publication Data for this title is available from the Library of Congress

ISBN 978-1-64411-400-1 (print)
ISBN 978-1-64411-401-8 (ebook)

Printed and bound in the United States by Lake Book Manufacturing, Inc.
The text stock is SFI certified. The Sustainable Forestry Initiative® program
promotes sustainable forest management.

10 9 8 7 6 5 4 3 2 1

Text design by Virginia Scott Bowman and layout by Debbie Glogover
This book was typeset in Garamond Premier Pro with Steagal and Avenir Next
and Gill Sans MT Pro used as display typefaces

To send correspondence to the author of this book, mail a first-class letter
to the author c/o Inner Traditions • Bear & Company, One Park Street,
Rochester, VT 05767, and we will forward the communication, or contact the
author directly at **www.themaleorgasm.com**.

Contents

Cannabis and Its Profound Effects on Male Intimacy

Dr. Pepper Hernandez

This highly informative book on cannabis and its positive influence on male sexual response provides the reader and first-time users a connoisseur's experience, an introduction to cannabis and its effect on the prostate gland and male sexuality. The idea that cannabis can play a part in the sexual stimulation of or act as an aphrodisiac for men has gained a good deal of momentum in the personal growth and medical communities. The science around the entourage effect or molecular synergy of cannabis and its ability to increase pleasure is documented in a growing number of scientific studies.

As a naturopathic doctor and transpersonal counselor, I founded the Cannabis Holistic Institute in Humboldt County in Northern California to teach others how to heal themselves with cannabis remedies and derivatives that respond holistically to the body, mind, and spirit. I've positioned myself to help others find their exact cannabis profile and application method for the desired outcome. I also currently write for more than half a dozen cannabis publications and consider myself a cannabis content creator.

Cliff is an advocate for the time-tested use of cannabis as a sexual sacrament, and he has developed several conference lecture series based on the cultural use of psychotropic plants, herbs, and other natural substances. In *Cannabis and Sexual Ecstasy for Men,* he has put together a very informative book that examines the potent, amplifying effect that cannabis has on sexual arousal, prostate gland sensitivity, and multiple orgasms. It is based on his personal experience with cannabis, his considerable research, and his expert interviews with people in the cannabis wellness sphere, as well as his work as the director of the San Francisco Cannabis Business Summit, which features cultivars, medical experts, and sex educators. This creative and original book is sure to become a wonderful addition to a growing list of cannabis health books.

DR. PEPPER HERNANDEZ, N.D., PH.D., C.T.C., C.N.H.P., N.H.C., is a board-certified holistic health practitioner and an award-winning doctor of holistic naturopathic medicine. She is the founder and CEO of the Cannabis Holistic Institute in Humboldt County in California. She is also an educator of health and wellness and an advocate, researcher, and author who has written for numerous publications and lectured internationally on the subject of cannabis and health.

https://www.drpepperhernandez.com

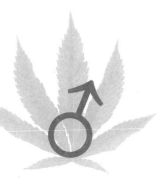

A Sexual Revolution for Men

It starts as a quivering deep inside of you. It makes your thighs tremble and your muscles contract in a very pleasurable way. It tightens up the way your penis would when fully erect and you are overaroused. It feels like a pressure inside of you. You can feel it rise up to your core, all muscles tightening at once . . . your temples shaking—that's how deep into your core this is reaching . . . and then it releases. You feel an extreme rush of endorphins and feel good chemicals, a warmth all over your body. You can barely think, just lay there in an ecstasy and a stupor as wave after wave of pleasure courses through you and all over you.

ANONYMOUS DESCRIPTION OF
A PROSTATE-CENTERED ORGASM FROM REDDIT

Across the United States and in countries where cannabis is legal, a growing revolution in male sexual pleasure is taking place. Men who ingest or smoke a small amount of marijuana and apply a simple internal massage are experiencing not just one but multiple orgasms, similar to what sexually active women have encountered for centuries. Intensely pleasurable, these orgasms produce no ejaculation, require no recovery period, and flow over the body in unrestricted convulsive waves.

At the root of this pleasure is the male G-spot, or prostate gland, a small walnut-sized organ that sits inside the lower abdomen just above the anal canal and below the bladder. The health and vitality of the prostate are essential to a man's sexual wellness. When the gland is irritated, inflamed, or affected with disease, the simple act of achieving an erection or ejaculation is nearly impossible. A healthy prostate can mean a comfortable release of urine, firm sustained erections, and when excited, multiple orgasms. There's even growing evidence that the prostate may secrete important hormones that contribute to overall male wellness. But many men are unaware of this organ's importance in their overall health, and most are unaware of its role in providing sexual gratification.

The catalyst behind this pleasure are cannabinoids, a group of chemical compounds found in cannabis that relax the mind and body, sensitize the genitals, and arouse the prostate gland, which triggers spasms we recognize as an orgasm. Cannabis has been called the "natural Viagra," and this is good news for men.

The first derivatives of cannabis are found at the dawn of civilized man. They emerged from Asia more than five thousand years ago and were prized for their medicinal purposes by the Chinese and Egyptians. Around the same time, the Hindus were cultivating the plant as an aphrodisiac. It was valued for its ability to rouse the male and female libido by increasing genital sensitivity while enhancing sexual pleasure. Temples dedicated to

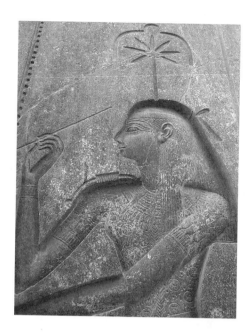

Cannabis above the goddess Seshat at Luxor Temple. Photo by Jon Bodsworth.

Lord Shiva, a god often associated with cannabis, are scattered throughout India and depict tantric yoga devotees who, through ritualistic consumption of a cannabis-infused drink called bhang, fueled their lusty gatherings for days.

This plant entheogen has not gone unnoticed by a growing group of sex educators, therapists, and health care professionals who advocate its use to reduce anxiety and boost intimacy. With its fast-acting psychoactive composition, a burgeoning industry of cultivators are developing new "sexy" cannabis strains that can act as an aphrodisiac and trigger heightened sexual arousal. For men, cannabis can increase blood flow and open neural pathways to the brain, sensitizing the prostate gland and the surrounding tissue. When using cannabis, men have reported having new types of orgasms of significant intensity and duration that affect the anus, colon, and prostate.

A JOURNEY OF SELF-DISCOVERY

Although this book is filled with practical advice on the cultivation of male multiple orgasms, it also chronicles my personal journey and sexual awakening. In May of 2019, I discovered that small doses of specific cannabis strains produced a level of intense sexual arousal that shocked and surprised me. After experimenting with various "sexy" strains of cannabis designed to raise arousal, I researched the phenomenon. Oddly, there is little in the way of reliable historical information on cannabis and its effects on sexual pleasure.

In the late 1980s, at the height of the cultural unrest in the United States, we got a sense of cannabis's health and aphrodisiac possibilities from rogue authors Robert Anton Wilson, Timothy Leary, and Terence McKenna, but it was too early to acknowledge the plant's possible benefits. Thankfully, through legalization, new research has opened us to the incredible wellness benefits of cannabis. As the former program director for the San Francisco Cannabis Business Summit, I compiled data on the latest applications of hundreds of new products with cannabinoids (THC and CBD) entering the market. However, my investigation turned up very little for us guys.

Male multiple orgasms are not a new phenomenon. There are men's groups and an industry filled with prostate massagers and techniques used to trigger orgasmic spasms known as multiple male orgasms. But for most men, multiple orgasms are elusive and practically impossible to achieve by just massaging the prostate. Health care professionals and sex educators are still in the dark on prostate-centered male multiple orgasms, but the reported results are startling. In one case, published in a medical journal, a sixty-three-year-old man who was using an antibiotic to relieve a condition of the prostate gland went to his doctor because he was experiencing multiple orgasms with such frequency that he couldn't perform his regular daily routines. So it appears that under the right conditions, a small number of men can have multiple prostate orgasms.

Although it is known that cannabis activates our pleasure centers in a methodology that reshapes our understanding of the human brain, our overall knowledge of cannabis, including its unique properties and how it profoundly benefits us, is in its infancy. As it becomes more available, this plant medicine, a natural aphrodisiac, can provide new levels of sexual pleasure for all. There's also a spiritual component to cannabis use and male multiple orgasms that is rarely reported. I discovered it at one point in my exploration, when I began having shifts in conscious awareness while consumed with overwhelming sensations.

In late 2019, I set out to chronicle my encounters, and this book represents a primer for men and women who are curious about a new and powerful method of increasing sexual pleasure. Every man and woman who has reached a level of sexual maturity deserves this orgasmic experience. In a manner of speaking, if you have this anatomy, it's your birthright to enjoy it!

HOW TO USE THIS BOOK

I strongly urge you to read through the entire book before actually trying the approaches detailed in later chapters. You should understand how your prostate functions as a sex organ, its relationship to the penis during sex, and how cannabis activates the gland before you attempt to achieve multiple orgasms.

The following chapters offer a fresh look at male sexual pleasure, including prostate orgasms, and cover the following areas:

Male orgasm and the prostate gland. It all starts with this amazing gland and its intricate connection to male sexual gratification. You'll learn how the prostate functions, what your doctor never told you about its importance in your overall sexual health, and why you must do everything you can to maintain its optimal wellness. Considered the male G-spot (or P-spot), this master gland is responsible for your sexual health and powerful male multiple orgasms. You'll discover suggestions for supplements and a lifestyle that can ensure a healthy organ and a lifetime of sexual pleasure. You'll also learn how lifestyle choices, including poor diet, excessive alcohol consumption, and lack of exercise can negatively affect your prostate and cause a declining libido (sexual desire).

Male multiple orgasms. Throughout this book, you'll learn about the anatomy of male multiple orgasms, how they're different from ejaculatory orgasms, and what role the prostate gland plays in achieving them. You'll discover an industry dedicated to stimulating the prostate gland through massage devices and why most of these appliances can damage the prostate.

Cannabis as a sexual catalyst. Many of us have experimented with cannabis and enjoy the passive sensations, pain relief, and feeling of well-being it can produce. But times have changed, and over the past decade, plant geneticists have developed a wide variety of cannabis strains that increase sexual arousal—the key to male orgasm. You'll discover how to incorporate small amounts of cannabis to enhance prostate sensitivity and produce multiple orgasms.

Self (sensual)-exploration. After decades, perhaps centuries, of misunderstanding, shame, and guilt surrounding male sexual self-exploration in most Western civilizations, men are now free to discover their bodies and the prostate gland, a new erogenous zone.

Resources. In this final section, you'll discover resources with the latest information on male sexuality and prostate wellness, cannabis arousal strains, cannabis tourism, cannabis and sex, and home-growing cannabis, as well as articles on the best prostate massagers on the market and vitamin and herbal supplements that can increase health and nerve function.

Until recently, only women were able to achieve multiple orgasms. Now—with a little patience—men, too, can experience, sustain, and repeat earth-shaking orgasms. Having robust, repeatable orgasms is not only highly pleasurable but also crucial for maintaining a high level of wellness in men twenty to eighty years old and beyond. Journey with me to uncover how to enhance your sexual pleasure exponentially.

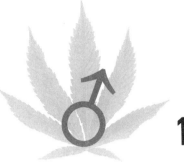

1

Who Is the Multiorgasmic Man?

Expressing the Full Measure of Your Sexuality

Exhaling, I began to shake uncontrollably as another spasm passed over me. But this wasn't the end of the experience, and sensing another orgasm tickling my prostate, I released into the intense sensation with a loud groan. This was something entirely new. There was something in the cannabis that had aroused me sexuality so that I could have a number of orgasms.

A FIRST-TIME USER OF CANNABIS WITH A
PROSTATE MASSAGER POSTED ON
THE ANEROS FORUM

An orgasm is one of the most pleasurable sexual activities we experience, and from our youth to our senior years, men will seek this ultimate gratification through masturbation or sexual intercourse. It's in our wiring to pursue orgasms not only because they feel good but also because they play an essential role in sustaining optimal wellness by releasing beneficial hormones like oxytocin into our system. When we ejaculate, a potent cocktail of chemicals is released into the bloodstream, making us temporarily tired or sleepy. Having an orgasm also appears to be a survival mechanism designed to boost the immune system and improve circulation to the reproductive organs. So, if a single orgasm is good for us, could having more than one in a single session be even better?

Most of us grew up discovering sex through masturbation. Although this self-pleasuring act relieved the sexual tension we experienced, as we matured and began to have sexual encounters, it quickly became apparent that women were entirely different in their ability to have not just one, but waves of orgasms. Until recently, it was thought that when a man masturbates or has sexual intercourse, he is able to ejaculate and orgasm once and then is forced to wait before arousing himself again to repeat the process. Not so for women, who, for hundreds of years, have chronicled their sexual awakenings in numerous books and articles and described a full range of orgasmic sensations, their effects, and how they were unleashed by masturbating, sexual intercourse, or through other methods of sexual stimulation. Under the right conditions, women can reach the levels of arousal that result in not one but multiple orgasms without a rest period that last for several minutes or significantly longer, a condition very few men can duplicate. These multiorgasmic women have fascinated men for centuries, and our own inability to sustain arousal long enough to achieve more than one orgasm at a time has been a source of frustration.

The male orgasm starts with the sensations he feels in his penis. As sexual arousal continues to build, he develops an erection and will eventually ejaculate and experience the pleasure of an orgasm. But recent discoveries reveal that the penis is just one source of stimulation that leads to an orgasm. The sex organ, or in this case sex gland, that triggers an orgasm is the prostate. Located within the lower abdomen, just below the bladder and above the anal canal, the prostate gland is a small walnut-sized organ. The actions of masturbation or sexual intercourse stimulate the prostate and trigger the release of semen. During an orgasm, the prostate has a muscular spasm that pushes seminal ejaculate and sperm from the testicles into the urethra and out through the penis. This single orgasm, depending on the age of the individual, is not immediately repeatable without a recovery period.

Most of us don't think of the prostate as a sex organ. We're only reminded of its presence when we develop an infection like prostatitis (inflammation of the gland), have a benign or cancerous growth and must seek treatment, or when it swells in our later years, pinching the urethra and reducing the flow of urine. Doctors typically recommend antibiotics to reduce the size of the gland if the swelling is caused by an infection, and natural remedies like pumpkin seeds and saw palmetto along with diet change appear to help. In chronic conditions, surgery may offer some relief, but this is only a temporary remedy.

Over time, other therapies, including prostate massage, have moved to the top of the list. When the gland is massaged, accumulated fluid is forced into the urethra and passed out of the body when a man urinates. This "milking" procedure is done in a doctor's office or, with instructions, at home. This therapy requires the patient to push a finger into the rectum, and with directed strokes, massage the prostate, which sits a few inches above the anal canal.

In 1997, High Island Health (HIH), a company based in Houston, Texas, began marketing a series of prostate massagers based on patents by Japanese urologist Dr. Jiro Takashima. Made of medical-grade plastic, these small hands-free massagers anchor outside the rectum, fit inside the colon, and press up against the prostate. By tightening and relaxing the PC, or pubococcygeus muscle, of the pelvic floor, the device gently massages the prostate to reduce inflammation and return the prostate to its normal size. In a small percentage of cases, men reported a pleasurable side effect of this therapy: convulsive spasms of extreme pleasure capable of shaking the entire body, which in some cases lasted for hours.

As word began circulating about the coveted prostate orgasm, a handful of sex toy manufacturers released prostate stimulators in all shapes and sizes in an attempt to capture the market of sexually curious men. The most successful of these is Aneros, a spin-off from HIH, who, in 2003, rebranded their prostate massagers as sex devices for men. Thousands of curious men purchased these devices and visited the Aneros forum to support and discuss their growing awareness of their prostate and the elusive Super-O, or super orgasm, a term coined by an early Aneros experiencer.

But using the massager was not a guarantee of a multiorgasmic session. Most were left discouraged and unsatisfied with the occasional spasm or slight tingle, far from anything orgasmic. In response, manufacturers introduced electric stimulators in an attempt to batter the prostate into submission with vibration, which in most cases only served to desensitize the gland and frustrate the user, who wasted his money on a useless device.

ENTER THE SEXUAL SACRAMENT

Today, thanks to the growing legalization of cannabis, men can discover how this powerful aphrodisiac alters the body's vibratory rate, increasing sexual arousal, and—with the gentle stimulation from a prostate massager—provides the multiorgasmic experience they desire.

None of this would be possible without the chemical compound tetrahydrocannabinol, or THC, the psychoactive stimulant found in cannabis. THC is a powerful substance that affects the body, mind, and spirit in an orchestrated event that stimulates the prostate while opening direct pathways to the brain and higher guidance, or our intuition. The chemical ingredients suspend the mind from the daily noise of our busy lives, slowing it down while relaxing the nervous system to become receptive to the body's sensations. Early cultures understood the properties within this plant as a sexual stimulant and ingested or smoked it or applied it in a lotion to increase genital sensitivity and the intensity of their orgasms. In ancient Hindu texts, women described rubbing cannabis resin on their skin and genitals to increase sensitivity and sexual pleasure. It's not clear if men from this period experienced heightened sensitivity, or, for that matter, orgasms, from such a practice. Still, it appears that cannabis was an essential part of orgies to enhance sexuality during coitus, the act of sexual intercourse. Today, we're just beginning to rediscover the effects of cannabis on the sex organs.

A SEXUAL RENAISSANCE FOR MEN

Now that we understand that cannabis and its benefits on human sexuality have been with us down through the ages, let's put the multiorgasmic man into perspective. Medical science has just scratched the surface in describing the orgasm and its effects on the brain and body. What is coming to light are the profound effects an orgasm has for healing, aligning the mind/brain, and connecting with our higher guidance. Also, repeating orgasms may lead to what neuroscience refers to as neuroplasticity, or a rewiring of the brain. When we do something pleasurable and repeat it successfully, we change the brain's function in a manner that makes it easier to reproduce favorable results, in this case an orgasm.

Perhaps what's most exciting for men's sexuality is what I call "sexercising," a short series of techniques that aid in triggering waves of orgasms. Outlined in this book, this method cultivates multiple prostate orgasms into easily reproduced events that, with proper recovery time, can be enjoyed throughout the lifetime of any man in fair to good health. Combining small amounts of cannabis with the light stimulation of a massager trains the brain to recognize the prostate and opens new pathways by rewiring the nervous system. For the vast majority of men, experiencing a single event with multiple orgasms now becomes a regular activity that can be enjoyed one or two times a week.

This game changer propels men to the heights of sexual pleasure that women have enjoyed since the beginning of time. Prostate orgasms represent an evolution in male sexuality, and, by experiencing multiorgasms at greater and greater intensity, a man can elevate the sensation of a penile ejaculation and enter a new realm of pleasure. Though there are no studies on the intensity of these orgasms, I believe that with proper care and a period of recovery between sessions, regular practice can move one into experiencing orgasms that transcend "normal" states of awareness.

If ever there was a sexual revolution in the making, it's now, as more men can begin to enjoy their full sexual awakening. Through my own research and studies of other men who have described their experiences, I've discovered that the benefits of these orgasms are multifaceted. Successful sessions can release pent-up emotions, anxiety, and a host of other issues we face. The experience of a multiorgasmic release is so overwhelming for most that the act, in general, is taken over by the autonomic system. As the body spasms with powerful convulsions, toxins are released, and other benefits yet to be understood are experienced. With practice, men are no longer limited to a single orgasm and can now experience intense multiorgasmic bliss with or without the presence of a partner or spouse.

Welcome to the age of the multiorgasmic man.

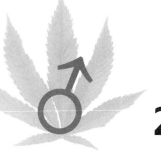

2

The Prostate Gland

The Center of Your Sexual Universe

When a man is engaged in a pleasurable sexual act, either through masturbation, releasing into an ejaculatory orgasm with a partner, or a multiple orgasmic episode such as the type highlighted in this book, the last thing he is thinking about is the function or condition of his prostate. It's only when he is confronted with the physical discomfort of prostatitis, an enlarged prostate, or benign prostatic hyperplasia (BPH), which restricts the flow of urine, or a diagnosis of prostate cancer that he considers the prostate and how it affects his life. Most men think of their penis as the center of their sexual universe, but it's the prostate gland that can deliver hours of intense sexual pleasure with or without a partner.

The prostate is a walnut-sized gland that sits inside the body about two to three inches beyond the anal canal, below the bladder and above the muscles of the pelvic floor. Most men discover their prostate when they visit the doctor for an annual physical exam and have their prostate palpitated to determine if there are any growths or abnormalities. The average prostate size for an adult male ranges from 15 cubic centimeters (0.9 cubic inch) to 30 cubic centimeters (1.8 cubic inches) and has the texture of a firm ripe plum or walnut shell. When aroused, the prostate will enlarge with seminal fluids that are released during ejaculation, making it firmer to the touch.

The prostate is regarded as a gland and not an organ because it secretes fluids during ejaculation that help the sperm survive the acidic environment of the vagina. It's also a muscle that contracts during sexual intercourse and forces semen out through the penis into the vagina and cervix, where egg fertilization and procreation take place. It's this prostate contraction that produces the deep sexual sensation of an orgasm, or "cumming," that feels so good. This is why the prostate is considered the male version of a woman's G-spot and when stimulated can produce an excep-

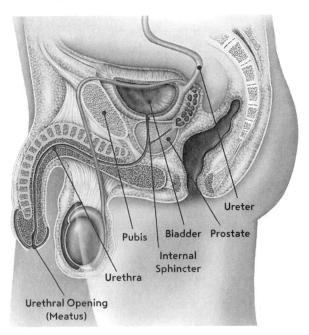

The prostate gland.

tionally strong sexual response and intense orgasms. This master gland also controls a group of nerves that lead directly to the penis and, when men are sexually aroused, signals it to swell with extra blood, producing an erection.

A VITAL SEX AND WELLNESS GLAND

Now that we understand the role the prostate plays in our sexuality, it should also be noted that this amazing gland performs a significant role in our general health too. In addition to signaling the release of blood to the penis during sex, it also releases 5-alpha-reductase.

The enzyme 5-alpha-reductase converts the hormone testosterone into dihydrotestosterone, or DHT, which is ten times more potent than regular testosterone. DHT is a male sex hormone that, when combined with testosterone, creates our sex drive. It is also important for general body and muscle growth and is what gives us our deeper (male) voice.

DHT and testosterone have mistakenly been targeted as the "guilty" hormones that contribute to prostate problems, but a body of new research is revealing that lifestyle choices may instead be at the center of this growing health crisis. High estrogen levels found in commercial meats, dairy foods, and body-care and household products appear to be leading contributors to lower testosterone and decreased prostate function. In general, processed foods that are high in sugar and fats can contribute to inflammation and problems of the prostate (prostatitis) and should be avoided. Beer and wine used in moderation appear to be fine, but overindulging can lead to negative prostate issues, including decreased function. I recommend avoiding all alcoholic beverages during sexual interactions, as they directly affect the body's ability to respond to the heightened arousal produced by the cannabis sacrament and decrease the prostate sensitivity that triggers an orgasm.

A sedentary lifestyle can also contribute to prostate problems, with lack of exercise and sitting for long hours the chief causes of a sluggish gland. Normal to moderate exercise is recommended for healthy sexuality, and activities as simple as walking three days a week can have the effect of normalizing the functions of the prostate and its ability to provide endless pleasure.

The content of this book is also good news for men of all ages, whether or not you're in a relationship. A healthy, functioning prostate can provide endless hours of sexual pleasure on levels of orgasmic intensity that will leave you breathless. Thankfully, this is not a one-off experience, and with short recovery periods, you can repeat these multiorgasmic sessions into an advanced age.

MULTIPLE ORGASMS, ERECTILE DYSFUNCTION, AND CANNABIS

Men with erectile dysfunction (ED), a condition that affects more than thirty million men, will be happy to learn that with or without a partner, an erection is not necessary to experience multiple prostate orgasms. With a new understanding that the penis is not the center of a sexual experience along with a healthy prostate gland sensitized with a "sexy" strain of cannabis, a massager, and a comfortable setting, any man can produce powerful orgasms. These types of orgasms have an additional benefit of increasing blood flow and nerve sensitivity within the prostate, which can support stronger erections during sexual intercourse. This may also lead health practitioners to recommend the use of cannabis and the program outlined in this book as a prostate recovery therapy to increase the health of the gland and normalize its functions.

Medical science has come to the realization that the prostate may be the cause of a number of the problems associated with ED. According to prostate.net, a website devoted to prostate health, having an enlarged prostate alone does not cause ED. However, scientists are still uncertain why BPH and its lower urinary tract symptoms are associated with ED. One idea concerns the sympathetic nervous system, which studies show is hyperactive in animals and men with BPH-associated urinary tract symptoms. Nerve fibers in the sympathetic nervous system transmit signals that have an impact on stress and stress-related symptoms. An increase in these signals may lead to overactivity in the sympathetic nervous system, which is associated with erectile problems. This confirms that the health of the prostate is critical for general wellness and male sexuality.

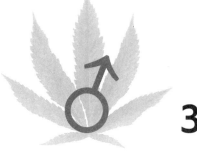

3

The Male G-Spot

Triggering the Multiorgasmic Experience

Most of us have heard of the G-spot: a place within a woman's vagina that when stimulated in a certain manner and in the right circumstances (environment, mood, psychoactive substances, etc.) is the key to achieving an earth-shattering vaginal orgasm. Named after Dr. Ernst Gräfenberg, the urologist who discovered it, the G-spot is a *scientifically researched* area that can give women incredible pleasure. It's identified as the female prostate and demonstrates traits and functions similar to the male prostate, which, when properly stimulated, can provide a multiorgasmic experience complete with ejaculating prostatic fluid. The male prostate gland, until recently, was just one in a group of sex organs responsible for producing an ejaculatory orgasm following an erection. Little did we know that when awakened it could give men incredible pleasure in durations lasting for hours. This is an area of male sexuality that must be researched more closely to understand more completely what men are experiencing. I've read extensively about the experiences of men who documented their orgasms and observed others who captured their intimate experiences on camera, and in each case it's plain to see that all were having spasms, convulsions, and different levels of intense pleasure unlike the simple penile orgasm.

What's an orgasm? *Merriam-Webster's Dictionary* defines it as follows:

1. A climax of sexual excitement, characterized by feelings of pleasure centered in the genitals and (in men) experienced as an accompaniment to ejaculation
2. Intense or paroxysmal excitement; *especially:* the rapid pleasurable release of neuromuscular tensions at the height of sexual arousal that is usually accompanied by the ejaculation of semen in the male and by vaginal contractions in the female

Before the discovery of the prostate orgasm, men were limited in their sexuality to only an ejaculatory orgasm, which was accomplished in stages.

In stage one, a man perceives something or someone that prompts sexual interest. That perception prompts the brain to send a signal down the spinal cord to the sex organs, causing an erection. The penis becomes erect, the scrotum is drawn up into the body, and muscles throughout the body increase in tension.

In stage two, known as the plateau, the body prepares for orgasm, muscle tension increases even more, and involuntary body movements, particularly in the pelvis, begin to take over. The heart rate increases and preejaculatory fluid is sent into the urethra to smooth the path for sperm.

Stage three, the orgasm, occurs in two phases: emission and ejaculation. In emission, the man reaches ejaculatory inevitability, the "point of no return." Semen is deposited near the top of the urethra, ready for ejaculation. Combing the fluid from the prostate and seminal vessels, an ejaculation occurs in a series of rapid-fire contractions of the penile muscles, the prostate, and the base of the anus.

In stage four, resolution and refraction, the penis begins to lose its erection. About half of the erection is lost immediately, and the rest fades soon after. Men usually must undergo a refractory period, or recovery phase, during which they cannot achieve another erection. In an eighteen-year-old, this is typically less than fifteen minutes. In elderly men, it can be up to ten to twenty hours. The average refractory period is about half an hour.

Prostate orgasms are uniquely different and contain no resolution and refraction periods, opening continual waves of highly pleasurable intense orgasms that, under the right conditions, can last for several hours.

AWAKENING THE PROSTATE

Some men, those who have experience with prostate stimulation or anal play, are able to attain the Super-O, or multiple orgasms, immediately with a massager. For others, achieving any type of prostate orgasm will require a learning and training period. During this time, through practice, a man and his body will discover that they may be capable of producing and experiencing unique, pleasurable sensations in greater amounts than they ever had before. This so-called journey to the Super-O stands alone as a singular and extremely personal time in a man's life. Each man has his own unique anatomy, and through practice he can begin to understand how the body, mind, and spirit work together to reach incredible heights of pleasure.

By using a massager along with a number of preparatory steps, men can achieve overwhelmingly strong nonejaculatory orgasms that involve full-body waves of pleasure and sensory reactions. This new type of orgasm transcends the sexual pleasure men normally achieve through the penis, by stimulating the prostate gland directly, which, through its connection to the nervous system, delivers orgasms of great intensity. Most of the men who achieve the Super-O experience a variety of sensations that can only be categorized as transcendent. They include the following:

- Intense pleasure throughout the pelvic region, particularly the prostate, rectum, and surrounding muscles
- Loss of a sense of reality
- Strong emotional responses
- Flashes of color (optical activity in the brain)
- Large muscle contractions
- A strong sense of ejaculation (with no emission)
- Protracted involuntary vocalizations (roars and screams)
- Pleasant convolutions
- Pronounced deep and staccato pelvic thrusting or writhing
- A sense of soulful release and relief
- A sense of self-redefinition
- An energized feeling immediately following orgasm and being ready for more

What makes prostate orgasms highly pleasurable is the nonejaculatory, zero-resolution aspect that is required when you have a penis-centered orgasm. Multiple orgasms are possible because your body never falls from a highly aroused state, and you're effectively staying in the plateau phase between orgasms. The duration of a Super-O may be several seconds to a minute or longer than a traditional orgasm and reached in waves. Super-Os come in all shapes and sizes. Some are small, others are large; they can be single orgasms or clustered together and centered in single or multiple areas. What's fascinating is some are very intense while others are on the light side, but overall the experience is one of surging pleasure in waves that leaves one in a blissful yet energized state.

It should be noted that multiple prostate orgasms are personal and different for each man and can elicit an emotional release from the deepest level of our being. Men have reported sobbing uncontrollably after these intense orgasms and feeling vulnerable because their normal awareness has shifted.

In some reports, men had out-of-body experiences and in the throes of multiple orgasms were delivered into altered states, which required the body's autonomic systems to effectively take over. On this unconscious level, the body moves in anticipation of an oncoming orgasm, experiences it, and then after a brief rest period, contracts muscles in the pelvis floor or another part of the body to deliver stimulation to produce another orgasm. In videos featured on YouTube, a small number of men, under the title of Prostate Orgasms, can be seen in various orgasmic states during a session. In each example there appears to be a powerful pleasure wave action that takes place and a buildup, perhaps smaller orgasms that reach a peak and in some cases trigger a convulsive reaction (intense concluding orgasm), which is then repeated. This is different for each man, and most appear possessed as powerful convulsive orgasms shake their bodies—they are seen groaning in pleasure in a semiconscious state of extreme arousal. What's fascinating and a wonderful

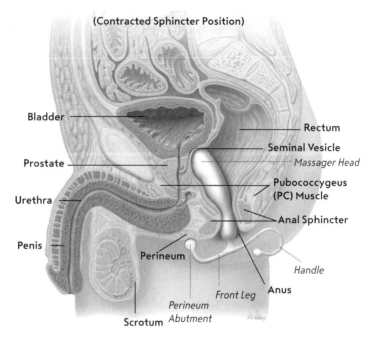

The prostate massager as it connects with the prostate gland.

experience for a man is that the cycle can repeat itself for a number of hours, which eventually produces physical and mental exhaustion, and the experiencer may fall asleep or decide to end the session.

As hot as multiple orgasms appear, some men can run into problems. As documented in a recent scientific research paper titled "Prostate-Induced Orgasms: A Concise Review Illustrated with a Highly Relevant Case Study," a sixty-three-year old man confessed that he had become addicted to his multiple orgasmic sessions. The unnamed man was healthy, with a normal prostate and high sex drive. He purchased a prostate stimulator to massage his tender prostate after an infection. Combined with his daily tadalafil prescription (an ED and urinary tract infection drug), the sex toy made the infection go away. But he also began having extreme orgasms of the Super-O category. He felt them everywhere—his penis, his anus, his pelvis, and his perineum (the place between the anus and the scrotum). According to the paper, "the subject found that whilst the orgasms were extremely enjoyable at the time, he could easily spend too much time experiencing them. Further, he had an old neck injury which flared up in association with some neck spasm at orgasm whilst lying prone. It has proved difficult to stop experiencing these orgasms and 'unwire' himself back to normal." The paper continues to say that the man stopped using his prostate massager and went back to having regular sexual relations with his wife and occasionally masturbating.

It should also be noted that the prostate orgasm represents an evolution in understanding male sexuality, and there is a great deal of research that must be conducted to understand the effects on the brain and body. This precious gift is a new awakening for men on multiple levels, and I believe it is designed to provide us with a direct line of communication to our higher guidance—that little voice in our head that appears when we need advice, often referred to as our intuition or our higher self. During a multiple orgasm session, the prostate may also release precious healing hormones and clear nerve synapses in the spinal column and brain that are vital to optimal health and wellness.

So stigmatizing this experience by labeling it as a problem or an abusive event could potentially be taking away an activity that men need in their lives to help them cope and to rejoice in who they are as human beings. And although the example above points out the subject's inability to control these extreme orgasms, there are ways to regulate them and prevent them from becoming addictive. (Read about controlling your orgasms in chapter 8, where I provide methods for stopping the flow of orgasms and other techniques when you have to end a session. Chapter 11 "Multiple Orgasms, Obsession, and Addiction" provides strategies to prevent obsession and addiction.)

While this new sexual revolution seems exciting to consider, the sad truth is that only a small percentage of men are able to achieve Super-Os just by using a prostate massage device. Hundreds or perhaps thousands of men who have purchased a massager have spent hours carefully following the directions outlined in user forums, but even with rigorous adherence to the prostate stimulating techniques, they rarely if ever achieve multiple orgasms.

There are numerous reports from men who could not feel any sensations and were left frustrated and disappointed because they were not able to achieve multiple orgasms or any sexual stimulation at all. I spent years using a massager, seeking to have the ultimate sexual experience, but having achieved few results I eventually became frustrated and disinterested as well.

It is important to note here that while the prostate massager is an important tool in stimulating the gland and contributes to the overall multiorgasmic experience, there's a subtle rewiring of the brain—called neuroplasticity—that must take place before the prostate will react to stimulation. This rewiring involves training the brain to open new neural pathways to connect the prostate, brain, and higher guidance. While this is certainly possible for those so inclined, the average man seeking this kind of orgasm has another option: he can include the stimulant cannabis, which will lift his state of arousal while activating and sensitizing the prostate to produce this new type of orgasmic experience. When cannabis is used with the massager it removes the need for a time-consuming and frustrating trial-and-error period of rewiring the prostate. As you'll read in the next chapter, cannabis has the distinct ability to deliver the high level of arousal, relaxed body, and host of other pleasurable effects that are important in achieving multiple orgasms.

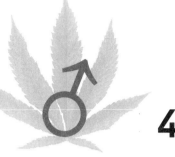

4

The Cannabis Connection

A Divine Sexual Sacrament for Men

When I came, I went temporarily deaf with ecstasy.
COMMENT ON THE ANEROS FORUM

The catalyst for male sexual awakening outlined in this book is cannabis. Without the chemical compounds in this plant, there would be no means to elevate arousal and suspend the active mind long enough to allow for multiple orgasms. In numerous studies, men who incorporated cannabis into their sexual activities began to experience not one but multiple waves of orgasms, which in some cases lasted for more than an hour. The key to these orgasms is sustained stimulation, a sensation that is different for each man. When the prostate gland was not sufficiently sensitized, or there were indications of prostatitis, the increased arousal wasn't enough to trigger a prostate orgasm. But through repeated use of the prostate massager in combination with cannabis, subjects were eventually able to rejuvenate the prostate and achieve orgasms of varying intensity.

Throughout this book, I will emphasize the importance of

microdosing cannabis to trigger an orgasmic response centered in the prostate gland. This consumption method is usually enough to sensitize the delicate nerves within the prostate to react to the slightest stimulation and open the body and brain to the effects of heightened arousal. This technique is readily embraced by men who are light or infrequent users of cannabis but may be an issue for those who consume daily for pleasure or health conditions. If you're using marijuana to experience "couch lock," where you've shifted into a state of brain fog or numbing out, you'll need to dial it down to a level that awakens the prostate. You'll know where you need to be when you're able to feel the tickling sensations of the prostate massager as it gently rubs against the gland. In some cases, heavy cannabis users may require a short period of abstaining from the plant to reactivate synaptic sensitivity. Chapter 8 provides step-by-step instructions on how to incorporate cannabis into a session that produces powerful full-body orgasms.

In this chapter, we'll learn about the effects of cannabis on male sexuality, various consumption methods, and the different "sexy" strains that promote heightened arousal, which leads to multiple orgasmic experiences.

CANNABINOIDS AND THEIR EFFECT ON SEXUAL AROUSAL

Cannabinoids are chemical compounds present in the resin of the *Cannabis sativa* plant, commonly called marijuana. These chemicals have a drug-like effect on the human central nervous system, leading to altered moods, pain relief, and other temporary changes. While cannabis produces more than one hundred different types of cannabinoids, the compounds noted for their ability to raise male sexual arousal are tetrahydrocannabinol (THC), cannabidiol (CBD), and terpenoids, or terpenes. Scientists recently discovered that the human body has a cannabinoid cell structure that they've named the endocannabinoid system, which influences physiological processes like appetite, mood, memory, and the libido. Currently, two primary endocannabinoid receptors have been identified and are known as CB_1 and CB_2. Within this system, cannabinoids mediate communication between various cells and systems in the human body through the interaction with the cannabinoid receptors.

CB_1 receptors work mainly on the brain and in the central and

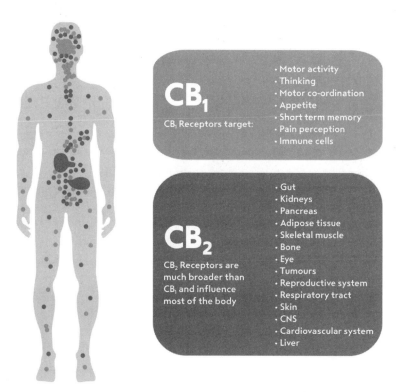

The human endocannabinoid system.
Diagram by WuttikitStudio.

peripheral nervous systems. In contrast, CB_2 receptors are found mostly in the immune and gastrointestinal system. When a cannabinoid attaches to these specific receptors, it triggers a series of changes in the way cells send signals to other cells. Scientists theorized that if we have this complex network of receptors, we must produce endogenous chemicals that also act as keys to the receptors' lock-like mechanism. It took awhile, but eventually they discovered anandamide, named after the Sanskrit term for divine joy because of the blissful sensations it produces. Anandamide is an endocannabinoid that functions as a neurotransmitter that sends chemical messages between nerve cells (neurons) throughout the nervous system. Anandamide is found in nearly all tissues in a wide range of animals and has also been found in plants and chocolate.

THC Cannabinol

THC is the primary psychoactive component of the cannabis plant. In other words, THC is the primary agent responsible for creating the high associated with recreational cannabis use. This compound works, in part, by mimicking the effects of anandamide, which include sleeping- and eating-habit modulation, pain perception, and countless other bodily functions. THC is also essential for increasing a man's capacity to have multiple orgasms because of its ability to activate the nerves of the sex organs and the prostate gland to heighten arousal.

Some of the effects of THC include the following:

- Relaxation
- Reduced stress and anxiety
- Improved creativity
- Altered senses of sight, smell, and hearing

- Increased appetite
- Reduced aggression
- Heightened sexual arousal

CBD Cannabinol

CBD is one of the most beneficial cannabinoids in the cannabis plant and exists both in agricultural hemp and cannabis. While cannabinoids are present within several plants in nature, cannabis is the only plant known to contain CBD. CBD's medical benefits are profound and affect a growing list of neurological and physical conditions dramatically. Current research from the Cannabis Holistic Institute indicates that CBD may be useful in helping with the following:

- Pain (neuropathic, chronic, cancer-related, etc.)
- Epilepsy
- Multiple sclerosis (MS)
- Inflammation
- Psoriasis and acne
- Broken bones
- Depression
- Bacterial infections
- Diabetes
- Rheumatoid arthritis
- Nausea
- Anxiety
- Attention deficit hyperactivity disorder (ADHD)
- Substance abuse/withdrawal
- Heart disease
- Irritable bowel syndrome (IBS)

Terpene Cannabinol

Terpenes (pronounced tur-peens), or terpenoids, have recently entered the cannabinoid discussion and are essential in distinguishing the flavor and smell of cannabis flowers. Terpenes are the aromatic metabolites found in the female cannabis plant and are identified for their ability to amp up, change, or lower the intensity and duration of a cannabis strain's effects. We'll learn more about the effects and contributions of terpenes later in this book.

OLD WORLD USE OF CANNABIS

More than five thousand years ago, Indian physicians developed a holistic healing system for wellness they termed ayurveda. Based on natural, noninvasive therapy, ayurveda includes dozens of cannabis formulations reputed to produce long-lasting erections, delay ejaculation, and loosen inhibitions. In the esoteric Hindu Buddhist tradition known as Tantra, a mystical religion that prescribed meditation and yoga, practitioners drank bhang, a liquid made from cannabis, to produce a psychophysical experience that brought forth waves of pleasurable orgasms. These tantric rituals sought to prolong sexual union as long as possible, and sacred texts describe cannabis-assisted intercourse as lasting for several hours.

Carvings and paintings of couples in a variety of sexual tantric contortions fill the walls of numerous temples in India as an homage to Lord Shiva. Shiva, the god associated with cannabis and yoga, suggested using cannabis in meditation and yoga to achieve Nirvana, the union of body, mind, and higher spiritual connection. Tantric practitioners believe the human body contains energy systems consisting of nerves, heart, and spiritual elements linked to cosmic and nature-based energies. Tantra identifies the

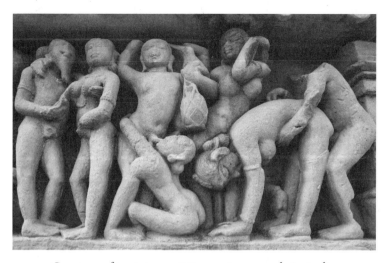

Carvings of tantric practitioners in a temple in India.
Photo by R. M. Nunes.

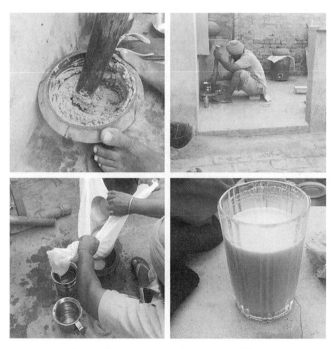

The modern process of preparing bhang.
Photos by Marcusprasad.

different male and female energy systems and unites these energies, creating "circuits," allowing participants to find new heights of intimacy and transcend egocentric consciousness.

Our knowledge of the effects and healing properties within this plant ally is limited. Until recently, unless prescribed for medical use, cannabis was considered an illegal narcotic and banned in much of the United States and other industrial countries. Our lack of research and understanding of the physiological, mental (and spiritual) effects of THC/CBD/terpenes has not stopped people from experimenting outside the clinical setting. An internet search for cannabis remedies will quickly reveal recipes for homemade tinctures, skin ointments, and suppositories created to deliver THC and CBD directly to the bloodstream. As cannabis continues to take hold in America, more companies are developing products that enhance genital sensitivity and provide the user with a heightened sense of awareness and arousal, leading to greater sexual pleasure. Foria Wellness, a California manufacturer that uses THC and CBD in its products, recently released a suppository designed with a low dose of THC to provide mild to moderate stimulation and aimed at women and men who enjoyed anal/prostate play.

CANNABIS AS A SACRAMENT

You'll notice that I use the term *sacred sexual sacrament* in describing cannabis, and although I'm not a religious person, the term has meaning for me. The cannabis sacrament provides an essential distinction from Western church doctrines. By eating a communion wafer, Christian devotees participate in a ritual that symbolically partakes of the body of Christ. Still, this sacrament also refers to a thing of mysterious and sacred significance, which is an essential distinction in cannabis.

I've studied several ancient cultures and, at a young age, aligned myself with the Hindu practices of meditation and yoga, which provide clarity of body, mind, and spirit. The Hindu sacraments can be regarded as an integral part of Dharma to develop the individual in every aspect. The person believing in rituals involves himself in worldly life and establishes a balance between mundane affairs and spiritual aspirations. In our use of cannabis as a sacred sexual sacrament, we ask that the plant open us to the full responsiveness of our sexuality and, through the orgasms we experience, align our being with spirit.

I want you to have a conscious awareness of what you're experiencing and how you got there through the connections delivered by this sacred plant. I believe that Old World cultures understood the impact that cannabis had on their psychospiritual sexuality and by integrating cannabis could connect with higher levels of consciousness. Today, a growing number of men are exploring the sacred sexual practices of the past and experiencing new levels of awakening through cannabis. Men using one or more of the latest designer arousal strains report profound orgasms and altered states of awareness. This form of male sexuality is so unique that institutions are beginning to take notice, and researchers are slowly coming around in their realization of the implications of male multiple orgasms.

CANNABIS FOR PROSTATE SENSITIVITY AND ORGASM

Cannabis is the ultimate male aphrodisiac: it has the ability to make us horny, stimulate our sex organs, and open a conduit directly to the brain, our master control center. It also lowers inhibitions and makes it easy to enjoy our sexuality, thereby opening us to experiencing multiple orgasms. The active cannabinoids in THC sensitize the prostate in the same manner intercourse or masturbation stimulates our penis, triggering a spasm. Cannabis acts on the body to arouse an orgasm to come faster and in layers that grow in strength and intensity. The multiple orgasmic session is prized by men who achieve it because it represents the most pleasurable experience they can have, transcending the pure ejaculatory orgasm by a magnitude that is off the charts.

More studies on the effects of THC on the brain are needed as we are still in the dark on just how it affects the nervous system, but for our needs, the stimulant in symphony with the prostate massager and a comfortable environment can deliver a profound orgasmic experience. With cannabis, whatever blocks, resistance, or reluctance we might encounter during ordinary consciousness is changed as our senses are magnified and released through an orgasm.

MICRODOSING FOR OPTIMUM EFFECT

The powerful effects of cannabis as an aphrodisiac have not gone unnoticed by several entrepreneurs, therapists, and authors who recommend it in their books, websites, blogs, seminars, and podcasts.

More research needs to be conducted on how cannabinoids work with the body to ignite an orgasm and open men to this amazing experience. I also believe that as more men experience multiple orgasms, plant geneticists will design faster-acting cannabis strains that produce different types of sexual arousal that will create signature orgasms of varying sensations and strengths.

In our quest for the multiorgasmic experience, we must respect the potent psychoactive stimulant THC and its effects on the prostate, brain, and nervous system. The goal is to consume just enough to enhance our perception and activate an arousal level where the slightest touch to the prostate triggers an orgasm. As many have discovered, overstimulation (getting too high) has the negative effect of numbing the body, perception, and delicate sensory receptors. Yet small doses or microdoses of cannabis stimulate a responsive prostate to activate the neural pathways responsible for orgasm. As the saying goes, less is more, and everyone from sexologists to noted authors suggest small doses to stimulate arousal. You don't want to get so intoxicated that you lose all sensation of having an orgasm or become unable to feel them to their fullest as they pass over your body. The one-hit method allows the body to amp up arousal and to consciously ride waves of orgasmic pleasure. In chapter 8, I recommend starting a session with a small amount, one to two hits from a vaporizer, joint, edible, and so on. Even better are the new line of products (vape pens, edibles, etc.) that deliver low THC doses, which provide the required stimulant for a sexual experience. Everyone is different, but in the end, the goal should not be to reach a level of couch lock, where you're giddy and numb and have little sense of your body. To birth the multiple orgasmic experience, the goal is to sensitize the body with a low dose of cannabis, turn up your arousal, and direct the energy to the prostate.

Adding the cannabis sacrament to a sexual encounter is the crucial ingredient that suspends your mind from its daily awareness, redirecting the focus to the body and opening neural pathways between the prostate, brain, and higher consciousness to create an orgasm. When you intend to have a multiorgasmic session, cannabis gently does the following:

- Heightens the senses, so you become more aware of your body
- Creates arousal, so you feel horny
- Helps to center your attention on the prostate and other sex organs
- Enhances the prostate massage sensation
- Triggers a response from the prostate
- Induces an orgasm
- Sensitizes the brain, so it experiences the orgasm and then after a break, repeats the event with a similar or more intense orgasm
- Cycles orgasms until the stimulation lessens or you end the session

In a growing number of men, the ability to have multiple orgasms represents a new sexual frontier, one that, until recently, was available only to a select few. Times have changed, and by introducing cannabis into a sexual encounter, men can now amplify their prostate sensitivity to react to the slightest touch, triggering an orgasm.

In the sexual experience I'm suggesting, a massager is only a tool used to "trip the switch," while cannabis opens a pathway through the nervous system to the brain, so you're plugged in and highly receptive to an orgasm. This new experience of delicate neuronal discharge must be approached carefully. You will not have this kind of orgasm if you're under the influence of alcohol, another psychoactive drug or stimulant, or are ill or have a degenerative disease that affects the nervous system.

Cannabis has so many beneficial effects for our sexuality. As I've studied its history and interviewed highly knowledgeable research investigators and authors, I've developed a deep appreciation for this medicinal plant and its effects on the human libido.

WHERE TO ACQUIRE CANNABIS AND THE "SEXY" STRAINS

There are different ways to legally obtain cannabis, depending on where you live and the laws that govern its use. In many countries where it is legal, you can visit a dispensary, have a delivery service provide strains that you've selected on the internet, or grow and harvest your own plants. Plant cultivation is the least desirable method to obtain the flower, as first-time growers face the challenge of producing quality plants that yield high levels of THC.

Access to cannabis varies widely among legalized countries and states and even among different cities. Recreationally legal states usually allow adults of a certain age to purchase cannabis from an approved store or delivery service. Medically legal states may require that a patient obtain a doctor's recommendation identified as a "rec" card to enter and purchase from a dispensary. To find a legal dispensary in your area, you can visit cannabis sites like Leafly, the Cannabist, and Allbud or simply download a phone app like Weedmaps.

As more states legalize the use of cannabis, the number of dispensaries will continue to grow along with varieties of strains. In California, there are individual and small chains of stores— similar to your local pharmacy—with good selections of strains and methods of consuming the herb. Many dispensaries carry seedlings that you can plant in a garden or transfer to pots for those interested in growing plants. If you're unfamiliar with the varieties of cannabis strains and their effects, most dispensaries have trained budtenders who are there to assist you with your selection. It's important to remember that no two people are the same, and if you're new to the effects of cannabis, you may need to sample different strains to discover which will deliver the desired results. In his book *The Passionate High,* sexologist Nick Karras suggests selecting from different strains and testing them. He says, "Since there are so many variants of each strain, I often advise first-time patients to visit the dispensary and tell the budtender that you are new to cannabis. Explain to them what your intentions are [arousal] and have them educate you on the variations within each strain. I then suggest purchasing a small amount of each of the three strains to sample. Keep the label from each and take notes as to how they affected you. You can then experiment with different environments like going for a walk, cooking dinner, or socializing with friends to help you discover what strain works best for you in different situations."

CANNABIS 101: SATIVA, INDICA, AND HYBRID STRAINS

Finding your unique cannabis balance is a journey of learning, exploration, and refinement. Getting too high teaches you about dosage, and feeling anxious or sleepy teaches you about the strain. The goal is to become aroused and to stimulate the prostate to produce an orgasm. The beautiful thing about cannabis is that even if you choose a strain that doesn't provide the stimulation you desire, the effects will wear off in a few hours.

It is also important to note that the fresher the flower, the stronger the effects. Buds that have been exposed to air for long periods have lost their potency and should be discarded. Keep your cannabis in an airtight container and a dark environment to preserve its freshness.

Ultimately you want to become a connoisseur of the "sexy" strains of cannabis and discover which flowers sustain arousal long enough to take you to the heights of an orgasm and then repeat the process to the degree that you experience orgasmic waves or multiple orgasms.

Sativa Strains

Cannabis sativa strains contain high levels of THC, which produce psychoactive and euphoric sensations. Strains that are high in sativa are suitable for people new to cannabis and for stimulating the prostate gland. Sativa strains are also ideal for boosting attention, awareness, alertness, and creativity and can arouse a sense of energy and motivation. They are also instrumental in treating depression, attention deficit, and mood disorders. Many people prefer to use a sativa strain during the daytime because of its positive, uplifting effect.

Indica Strains

Cannabis indica strains are high in CBD and produce a body high. They alleviate tension and sometimes facilitate sleep. Indicas are useful in treating muscle spasms, nausea, chronic pain, and tremors, as well as many other physical ailments. Some people prefer to use an indica strain later in the evening or at night since it makes sitting still or lying down seem heavenly. Indica may be beneficial in a sexual environment for those who have anxiety or are tense and need to relax to have a sexual experience. Others find this strain just makes them sleepy.

While the research on CBD looks promising for topical applications and wellness products, ingesting or smoking CBD produces little if any sexual stimulation for men and the prostate. For this and other reasons, hybrid strains with a mix of both sativa and indica are recommended. CBD oils and products offer perhaps the most significant new avenues for stimulating the prostate without the psychoactive effects. Currently, there are several products designed for women, which are noted for their ability to stimulate orgasm but seem to have little or no impact on male sexuality. For men, THC is the best method for the multiple orgasm pleasure we seek.

Hybrid Strains

With the growing legalization of cannabis in the United States, hybrid strains are on the rise, as plant geneticists continue to experiment with the effects and benefits of different strains. Hybrid strains are created by crossbreeding indica and sativa plants. Indica strains tend to relax the mind and body, while sativa components help to boost energy levels. Sativa-dominant hybrids enhance mood and motivation, but indica components can leave you tired and actually reduce or cancel out the sativa effect.

METHODS OF CONSUMING CANNABIS FOR OPTIMAL EFFECTS

When consuming a sexual sacrament, it's essential to keep in mind the ultimate goal: powerful, repeatable orgasms. To accomplish this, you must suspend the chatter of the mind and direct body stimulation to the prostate. The chemical compounds in THC are wondrous but extremely powerful, so the "less is more" theme should be your mantra. If you consume too much THC it can take you over the threshold, and if you consume too little, you won't feel enough stimulus to provide the prostate with the sensitivity needed for an orgasm.

Before you inhale or consume a cannabis product, you must set the intention to receive sexual pleasure. This will create the subtle environment needed to have a sexually charged session. As your body begins to experience tingling and other pleasurable sensations, your prostate will come online, triggering the start of an orgasmic session.

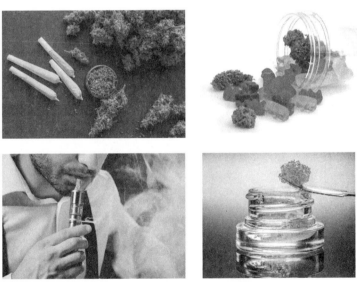

Cannabis is consumed in a variety of methods:
flower for smoking (by Dmitry Tishchenko), gummies
(by Mike Ledray), vaping (by Niromaks),
and concentrates (by 420MediaCo).

Smoking and Vaping

Smoking and vaping are the most widely used methods of consuming cannabis and are recommended for first-time users. Smoking consists of putting dry cannabis flower into a pipe or rolling a joint, lighting it up, and inhaling the smoke. Vaping involves inhaling heated oil through a vaporizing device, often referred to as an e-cigarette. Vaping can also refer to using a vaporizer to produce vapor from dried plant material. Some people believe vaping is safer than smoking because it doesn't involve inhaling smoke, but the reality is that very little is known about the health effects of vaping marijuana.

This approach to consumption delivers sensations within a few minutes and can last anywhere from thirty minutes to a couple of hours, depending on the strain and individual tolerance. You can also regulate the amount you consume and monitor the effects. Draw one good inhale into your lungs and hold it for as long as you can, then simply exhale. You should begin to feel something within ten to fifteen minutes. Remember, the goal is to take in a small dose to activate your body's sensual responses, so one hit on a joint, vaporizer, or pen is enough. Those of us who have been smoking for years will be tempted to take another draw—but resist. If you get too high, you will lose the body awareness and fall into the strong numbing effects of the THC. You want to feel high but also have a sense of your body. See chapter 8 for additional details on the multiorgasmic ritual and desired effects.

Edibles

Cannabis innovators are infusing foods and beverages—from baked goods to salad dressings—with THC. Since edibles pass through your digestive system, the effects take longer to kick in and tend to be stronger and longer lasting. As a result, it's typical for people to overdo it with edibles. Because you can overeat, the suggestion is to start with a small dose or a pinch-sized portion of an edible and then wait at least an hour after consumption to gauge the effects. The high from an edible typically lasts about four hours, but because the potency varies by batch, those new to cannabis should consider another method.

Tinctures

Cannabis tinctures are the compounds extracted from the plant and placed in alcohol- or glycerin-based solutions. Placed by dropper under the tongue or mixed into other liquids, these formulas provide fast-acting results and a more natural dosage control. They're available in many flavors, potencies, and cannabinoid profiles.

Dabbing

Dabbing is generally for the more experienced user. It consists of heating cannabis concentrate, which can pack a powerful stimulant, in a glass or metallic attachment and inhaling the vapors through a device such as a bong or a vape pen.

Topicals

Cannabis-infused lotions, salves, balms, and sprays are applied directly to the skin and can be effective remedies for the treatment of pain, swelling, and soreness. There is a growing list of sex lubes containing THC that have been reported to delay ejaculation and to increase the orgasmic response in women who use them directly on their genitals. Because of their lack of direct stimulation on the prostate, topicals are not recommended for men pursuing the multiorgasmic experience.

A FINAL NOTE ON THE SEXUAL SACRAMENTS

As a Northern California kid of the 1970s, I was introduced to cannabis, or "weed," in my teens and experimented with the strains that were available at the time. I can remember, with a smile, names like Maui Wowie, Thai Stick, and other strains that were low in potency and minimal in their effects but prized for their ability to shift the mind, numb the body, and on occasion amplify the user's awareness of their surroundings. Today, using cannabis as a sexual sacrament has made me aware of what a powerful gift it can be for men's sexual enlightenment. It truly is "plant medicine" in the form of a potent sexual stimulant that a man can now enjoy on his own or with a lover. This exceptional plant has the singular ability to open each of us up to our full sexual potential and the levels of healing, wellness, and connections to a higher awareness that are our birthright.

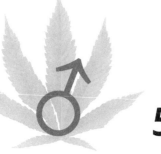

5

Sexually Stimulating Pot

How to Select Strains That Produce
Heightened States of Arousal

With more than one thousand cannabis strains developed across several decades, it's essential to select from the categories that provide high arousal and lead to more fulfilling sexual pleasure and orgasm. Marijuana affects each person differently, and no two people are alike. Strains recommended in articles, advertisements, or by friends may not work for you.

The best method of choosing a compatible plant is to do a little research before you purchase it. You'll need to experiment to discover which flowers are stimulating and produce the desired outcome. My recommendation for those seeking the ultimate reward—multiple orgasms and the ability to repeat the experience—is selecting among the strains that generate waves of arousal. In this chapter, I've provided a list of world-class cannabis strains noted for their ability to heighten touch and body sensitivity and open you to multiple orgasms. I've also developed a website, www.themaleorgasm.com, that supports the content in this book and provides the latest information and updates to assist you in all aspects of male sexual awakening and cannabis use.

A NOTE ON CONSUMPTION

Creating a setting that produces a sexual high and progresses to multiple orgasms requires an awareness of the amount of pot you consume. As mentioned earlier, most cannabis advocates and sex educators recommend small doses, with a single hit from a joint, bong, or pipe as your starting point. Wait for the effects to take hold before repeating the process. As your mind shifts and is slightly altered, your heightened body sensations will come online. At this point, any stimulation from touch, prostate devices, or visualization is amplified, allowing you to focus on your pleasure.

There are several methods for consuming cannabis listed in this book. Although vaping, edibles, and concentrates are popular, using the traditional smoking method allows you to get the full effect of the plant entheogen and the full spectrum of arousal. Once you've familiarized yourself with a "sexy" strain and can regularly achieve multiple orgasms, you can move on to other consumption methods.

If you consume cannabis daily or have a medical condition that requires you to smoke, vape, or ingest every few hours, you may have to dial it down for a week or more to allow the moderate to low THC "sexy" strains to work. Your higher tolerance blunts the effects of an arousal strain, masking the responsiveness and triggers that produce multiple orgasms. Remember, the goal is to elevate arousal (horniness), increase sensitivity, and direct your focus on the prostate gland. Concentrates, edibles, and other cannabis products with high levels of THC can create couch lock, numbing the senses.

TERPENES

No discussion on cannabis would be complete without a brief look at terpenes—how they work, and how they affect our sexual pleasure. Terpenes are hydrocarbon compounds found in cannabis and many other species of plants. Certain cannabis strains are incredibly rich in terpenes, and this gives them their pungent aromas. So you can thank terpenes for all the cannabis flavors and aromas you know and love. Whether you smoke cannabis flower, dab concentrates, or vaporize, terpenes are hard at work delivering tasty citrusy, diesel, woody, piney, skunky, coffee, spicy, herbal, or tropical flavors to your palate.

Growers seek to prioritize the hundreds of terpene compounds found in cannabis strains to enhance their flavor and scent, helping to improve the product's taste and marketed qualities. As cannabis consumption continues to grow worldwide, you will see terpene references added to the description of a plant's composition and quality, similar to the bouquets, or aromas, used to describe wine.

The following sections highlight some of the more notable and commonly found terpenes in cannabis.

Limonene
Limonene is recognizable for its zesty citrus fragrance, primarily lemon, but also orange, lime, and grapefruit. Limonene is found in the peels of these citrus fruits and in many varieties of cannabis. Along with myrcene, limonene is one of the most abundant terpenes in cannabis. It also has anti-inflammatory, antianxiety, antibacterial, and anticancer qualities.

Myrcene

Myrcene is one of the terpenes frequently found in cannabis. Its aroma is distinct, herbal, and citrusy. Myrcene appears to have a sedating effect, and studies have shown it as a potential muscle relaxant. In addition to sedative properties, myrcene may be an effective anti-inflammatory, and when combined with THC, contribute to couch lock, which is appreciated by recreational cannabis consumers.

Linalool

Linalool can be found in a variety of cannabis strains and contains a strong floral and spice aroma. Like myrcene, Linalool has several sedative properties, and studies suggest its natural ability to help with convulsions in seizures. Linalool's relaxing properties are also said to spread to being therapeutic in treatments of depression, anxiety, and stress.

Pinene

Pinene, true to its name, gives off a pine aroma. Like myrcene, studies have suggested that it has excellent potential as an anti-inflammatory. It also appears to be a bronchodilator, helping conditions like asthma. Additionally, strains with high concentrations of pinene were noted for their ability to help with memory.

Humulene

Humulene gives off an earthy aroma found in hops, one of the main ingredients in beer. Research on this terpene is limited, but it appears to be an appetite suppressant—not the kind of effect you would typically associate with marijuana. It is seen as having anti-inflammatory and antibacterial properties as well.

Caryophyllene

Caryophyllene's aroma is similarly woody but with more of a spicy scent than humulene. Found in black pepper, caryophyllene has been shown to have anti-inflammatory properties and is used to help treat duodenal ulcers.

Borneol

Borneol, with its distinct minty aroma, has been used in traditional medicine for a while. It is yet another terpene that can act as an anti-inflammatory, particularly for lung inflammation and neuropathic pain. It is also effective at repelling insects.

Terpineol

Terpineol's floral aroma is especially reminiscent of lilacs, and it can often be found in perfumes. Studies on terpineol tend to note its strong sedative effects. Combined with the scent, it's not unusual for terpineol to be implemented in aromatherapy.

THE ENTOURAGE EFFECT

Terpenes do more than provide flavor and aroma. They also support other cannabis molecules in producing physiological and cerebral effects. There is synergy between cannabinoids and terpenes, not to mention other secondary metabolites and phytochemicals. This synergy is called the entourage effect, and it's the reason terpenes have revealed themselves to be such a critical piece of the cannabis puzzle.

When multiple cannabis compounds are combined, their effects can be enhanced or altered. The flavors and psychoactive capacities may also be affected, creating distinct products with varying characteristics. In addition, the entourage effect of these combined compounds can have therapeutic effects, which arise from their ability to bind with naturally occurring endocannabinoid receptors in the brain and throughout the central nervous system.

The best example of the entourage effect is the interaction between CBD and THC. When taken on its own, THC gives users a "marijuana high"—the psychoactive effect that is commonly associated with cannabis use. It also may cause unwanted side effects, such as anxiety and paranoia. But when it is paired CBD, these side effects are reduced. CBD also enhances THC's potential medical benefits, such as pain and inflammation reduction, and adds some of its unique bonuses, like its possible antidepressant effects. The entourage effect may be one of the reasons why marijuana is such an effective medicine.

THE BEST SEX STRAINS

Although it's tempting to select one of your pot favorites to begin your sexual journey, I urge you to go through the list presented below and become familiar with the effects, types of sensations, and orgasms they produce. Later, you can move on to the newer advertised or "just released" arousal strains found in your state or country.

The following cannabis strains are time-tested, reviewed by thousands of men and women, produced by a growing number of cultivators, and readily available. When you're ready to purchase, choose from one or two strains from each type listed below:

- **Sativa dominant strains (example: Dream Queen, 70% sativa, 30% indica).** Sativa strains have cannabinoids and terpenes (limonene, for example) that usually offer a much more energetic and mind-driven high, leaving users more alert, uplifted, euphoric, and creative and with more stamina and a stronger desire to engage in any physical activity.

- **Indica dominant strains (example: Bubblegum Kush, 80% indica, 20% sativa).** Due to its high concentrations of myrcene, indica is responsible for a much stronger body high, resulting in complete relaxation, pain relief, sleep enhancement, and detachment from the body.

Both strains effectively relax you, lower your inhibitions, and raise your arousal to levels that trigger an orgasm. Enjoy the experience of sampling different strains while discovering which ones produce the desired sensation. Does a body high get you off better than a head high? I like to switch them up. One day it's a sativa-dominant strain, and then later in the week it's an indica for a quickie in the evening before bed.

AROUSAL STRAINS OF CANNABIS
BY PERCENTAGE

Strain	THC %	Sativa %	Indica %
Hindu Skunk	11–23	30	70
Jillybean	15.7	60	40
Granddaddy Purple	17–27	80	30
Trainwreck	18	90	10
Afghani Yumboldt	19	30	70
Dream Queen	19–22	70	30
Chem Dawg	19.5	45	55

Arousal Strains of Cannabis
by Percentage (*cont.*)

Strain	THC %	Sativa %	Indica %
Strawberry Cough	20	85	15
Girl Scout Cookies	20	40	60
Amnesia Haze	20–25	80	20
Sour Diesel	20–25	90	10
Bubblegum Kush	23	20	80
Super Silver Haze	23	70	30
XJ-13	23.8	50	50
Greek Crack	24	65	35
Jack Herer	24	55	45
Wedding Cake	25	40	60
Blue Dream	26.5	60	40
OG Kush	27	55	45
Northern Lights	33	10	90

Below is a short list of recommendations that can help you make educated and cost-effective decisions on selecting strains:

- Sampling loose cannabis flower can be expensive. When you visit the dispensary, consider selecting a "pre-roll," or joint, from a strain you'd like to sample. Pre-rolls can be a cost-effective method of selection when you're unsure about the effects of a flower.
- I've listed the strains to get you started exploring your sensuality and the ultimate goal of multiple orgasms. Please become familiar with them before moving on to others.

Once you've established a foundation of these strains, a casual internet search of arousal strains will turn up anywhere from 25 to 150 erotic blends.

- When you discover a strain that has you tingling with anticipation, or arouses you, take note of the effects in a notebook so you can build on your path to multiple-orgasm sessions. You can also transcribe notes from your audios (see chapter 9), so you have a list of your favorites. It's also a good idea to write down what didn't produce good results so you can save the expense of repeating undesirable purchases in the future.

WHERE TO PURCHASE CANNABIS

A growing list of online resources can help you locate stores, dispensaries, and delivery services in your area. Most legal states and countries have clusters of outlets in major cities and outlying suburbs. You should be aware of the legal age for consumption before you schedule a visit. In California, you must be twenty-one years of age or older to purchase cannabis. Also, not all dispensaries serve the general public. In states where there are a limited number of permits for selling cannabis products, you may find medical marijuana outlets that require a doctor's release. You can find details on how to obtain a release in the reference section of this book.

What is medical marijuana? The medicinal properties of cannabis come from its cannabinoids, the chemical compounds found naturally in the plant. States with medical marijuana programs have passed legislation through their government to legalize cannabis for medicinal use. These states have unique rules about who can grow, sell, and use medical cannabis. Each state runs its medical marijuana program independently. The state legislature governs everything from the cannabis formats that qualified patients can consume to the number of cannabis plants patients can grow at home. In many states where marijuana is recreationally legal, there are programs exclusive to medical marijuana patients that provide them with access to higher potency products, more generous cultivation allowances, discounts, and the ability to purchase more cannabis at one time. Those who qualify for these programs will also have access to the arousal strains highlighted in this book.

QUALIFYING FOR MEDICAL MARIJUANA

Despite federal law in the United States prohibiting the use of cannabis, there are many states with medical marijuana programs. These programs allow qualified patients to access cannabis from state-sanctioned dispensaries once a qualified medical professional certifies them.

Common Qualifying Conditions

Qualifying conditions are the diagnosable ailments for which patients may seek medical marijuana treatment. Each state has a different list of qualifying conditions. The following are commonly approved for the use of medical cannabis:

- Epilepsy and seizure disorders
- Cancer
- Multiple sclerosis (MS)

- HIV/AIDS
- Neurodegenerative disease
- Pain
- Nausea
- Post-traumatic stress disorder (PTSD)

THOUGHTS ON CANNABIS LEGALIZATION

As states across the nation begin to legalize adult-use cannabis, many may wonder how this affects medical cannabis dispensaries and cardholders. What does it mean to be a medical cannabis patient in a world where anyone can walk into a recreational dispensary, present their state ID, and legally purchase cannabis?

Many states with medical dispensaries offer lower-cost products for patients. Medical cards allow patients to access their medicine at a lower cost, making their health care more affordable and accessible.

Recreational shops are permitted to sell cannabis to anyone who is over the age of twenty-one. While this makes sense for the general populous, children who are also cannabis patients don't have access. Some medical cards allow those aged twenty and under to legally access cannabis medicine they need for their health care when treating cancer, epilepsy, or other ailments.

RESOURCES

Several useful online cannabis information websites and iPhone/Android apps are available, identifying the local or regional dispensaries carrying the most desirable strains. Below, I've provided a small list of them.

WEBSITES WITH DATABASE APPS

Weedmaps is a popular informational website that covers an international list of cannabis stores and dispensaries. Their powerful and up-to-date search database provides quick access to local and regional cannabis outlets.

Leafly is an excellent source for articles, research, and specific cannabis products. Its powerful search engine can help you locate dispensaries in your area that carry specific strains.

WEBSITES

Hail Mary Jane	Pot Guide
Wiki Leaf	Way of Leaf
Canna Connection	

PHONE APPS

High There	Eaze (marijuana delivery)	Duby
Weed Scale 4.20	Seamless	Best Bud
Grow Buddy		

6

Prostate Massage

Stimulating the Male G-Spot

There is no doubt about it—cannabis is a powerful aphrodisiac. Its compounds can effectively shift the body to a state of heightened arousal, provide a doorway to sexual pleasure, and turn a relaxed, private, and inviting environment into an erotic romp, producing unimaginable sensations and, in many cases, orgasms. But the prostate massager is the game changer. Once the body has become aroused and you're tingling with anticipation, the slightest touch, nudge, or rub of the prostate will induce an orgasmic reaction throughout the body.

While cannabis is the catalyst that sets an orgasm in motion by sensitizing the prostate, the hands-free prostate massager is an essential contributor to the process of achieving multiple orgasms. In this chapter, we'll discover how the massager works and the benefits of routine prostate stimulation. We'll also discuss the different types of massagers on the market and how to choose one to cultivate intense, full-bodied orgasms.

THE MODERN PROSTATE MASSAGER

Massaging the prostate gland has been practiced for thousands of years in India and China. It's also likely that the early Maya civilizations, who coveted sexuality as a sacred form of divine connection, were aware of the technique. Therapeutic prostate massage, also known as "prostate milking," is described in ancient Chinese texts and was prescribed to treat a wide variety of sexual dysfunctions and sexual stamina. The tantric masters attending China's dynastic emperors and their wives suggested prostate massage to maintain male fertility and as a form of sexual pleasure. While other Asian countries practiced this beneficial therapy, it also appears that Western medicine understood the importance the prostate played in male patients' health and prescribed massage as a remedy for various conditions. In 1890 the *Journal for the American Medical Association* (JAMA) recommended manual prostate massage therapy to relieve congestion caused by chronic prostatitis, infertility, and sexual problems.

It would take well over one hundred years after the JAMA article was published before the first hands-free massager would emerge that could stimulate the prostate and the surrounding areas of the pelvic floor and provide relief for men with chronic prostate infections and other conditions. As mentioned in chapter 1, Jiro Takashima, a Japanese urologist, developed and patented the first prostate massager, which in 1997 was manufactured and sold through HIH, a company based in Houston, Texas.

Takashima realized that a hands-free massager could increase blood flow to the gland while removing accumulated congestion and allowing for an easy and effective prostate massage. Regular therapeutic prostate massage shrinks an enlarged pros-

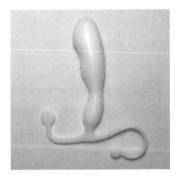

Aneros Helix prostate massager.

tate, decreases pressure on the urethra, and restores proper bladder function. He also recognized the benefits of Asian medicine and designed components into his massager that allowed the user to apply pressure directly on the perineum (a pressure point located in the space between the anus and scrotum). The massager was first sold to medical professionals for their patients. Takashima soon discovered that some men were reporting extraordinary sensations, and in a growing number of cases, intense orgasms. Shortly after, HIH rebranded the massagers under the company name Aneros.

The genius behind the Aneros massager is its shape. Composed of medical-grade plastic and anatomically designed to lie directly on the prostate gland, the device is hands-free and composed of four primary parts:

1. The massager's body comprises a head and stem, each constructed to pivot within the anal canal and colon. The head section nuzzles against the prostate and applies just enough pressure for an effective hands-free massage controlled entirely by anal sphincter and PC muscle contractions. The stem section is tapered to rest in the anal canal, which in itself is highly erogenous. Note that as your body

awakens to the stimulation, you may find that you can have exquisite anal orgasms that command your attention.

2. The perineum tab provides an external prostate massage by pressing up against the perineum and acting as a pivot point to drive the massaging action inside the rectum. This unique design is centered on a key pressure point for an important meridian, an area known for centuries in Asia to increase arousal when stimulated.

3. The kundalini tab (on the larger Progasm model) massages the acupressure point between the buttocks and sends stimulation up the spine.

4. The handle is used to insert and remove the massager and keeps the device from slipping into the colon, thus providing a hands-free massage.*

Despite the differences in physical characteristics, the prostate gland's location in approximately 98 percent of men is located two to three inches inside the anus. The Aneros massager ranges from three and a half to over five inches in length with varying thicknesses and conforms to different body configurations. Many men have reported positive results with a small group of Aneros massagers that have now set the standard for massagers worldwide. These include the Helix and Eupho models and the SGX classic. Every man is different, and you may find other models of Aneros more to your liking.

You may also find that a larger massager delivers the pleasure you're seeking. Many men report different types of orgasms

---

*Aneros has recently released the Trident series of massagers with redesigned tabs that contact the perineum and prostate in a more direct method.

depending on the shape of the device. If, for instance, you're using an Aneros Helix, one of my favorites, the design of the massager features a bulbous head, which pushes the prostate at different contact points, creating an immediate reaction and a strong orgasmic response. A longer and thinner massager like the Aneros Eupho gently taps and massages the prostate, tickling the gland while producing an orgasm that is repeated in small waves. Other massagers can trigger different types of orgasmic sensations, and you may find, depending on your mood, that having a selection of massagers on hand can add to the excitement of a session.

ANEROS VS. COMPETITOR MASSAGERS

Although there are countless other prostate massagers on the market, I am focusing on the Aneros line of products here because none of the others have the time-tested stamp of approval or the correct design to produce multiple orgasms as quickly and as effectively as the Aneros massagers do. It's also important to note that other massagers come in all shapes and sizes but are not necessarily anatomically correct, which can make them dangerous and uncomfortable to use.

An internet search for prostate massagers will return pages of stimulators that look more like butt plugs and dildos than a device for stimulating the gland. The best reviewed massagers are small (about the length of a long finger) and designed to contact the prostate, so as with cannabis, the idea that less is more should be a consideration when choosing a massager. A word of caution here: Because manufacturers are often in a rush to enter the lucrative market of male sex toys, many devices are created too quickly and without attention to detail. This means that massagers don't always conform to the interior of the colon, surrounding tissue, or the prostate, and this puts users at risk. In fact, the key reason I am shamelessly promoting the Aneros massager is the simple fact that it was designed by a practicing urologist, a physician intimately aware of the prostate and the surrounding organs in the lower abdomen and pelvis and their functions.

HOW THE MASSAGER WORKS

The Aneros massager is moved entirely by the muscles in the pelvic floor, but primarily by your anal sphincter. These muscles are naturally active during sexual stimulation and orgasm, and their contractions are a necessary component to your experience of sexual pleasure. Massagers exploit this automatic muscular activity to provide stimulation of many of your most sexually sensitive areas. The pulsing of the muscles causes the massager to press and pivot on your perineum and to rub your prostate, anus, and rectum. Remember: choose a massager designed to conform naturally to the prostate.

As the compounds in cannabis take effect, this rubbing and contracting become involuntary (they take off by themselves), and as the pleasure mounts, you begin to have orgasms. The massager gently stimulates your prostate, perineum, rectum, and anus, creating deep pleasure, probably unlike what you have felt before. The motion can range from very subtle, where you aren't sure it is moving, to perceptible small-distance stroking and broad, bold strokes that feel like receptive intercourse. All have their distinct flavor of pleasure. A detailed review of prostate massagers can be found on the author's website, www.themaleorgasm.com. Some massagers may also significantly improve partnered sex. Your erec-

RELAXED SPHINCTER

Prostate

Cowper's Gland

Bulb

Abutment

Head

Relaxed
Sphincter

CONTRACTED SPHINCTER

Prostate is squeezed
between the head
and the abutment

Cowper's Gland
is pushed up

Bulb is
pushed up

Abutment

Head

Contracted
Sphincter

*With the massager inserted, the PC muscles are contracted,
pulling the head of the device against the prostate gland.*

tions will be stronger, your ability to control your orgasms will be enhanced, and your general sensuousness will be increased.

WHAT DO MALE MULTIPLE ORGASMS FEEL LIKE?

The combination of the cannabis sacrament, a massager, and a comfortable setting can set in motion a sexual event unlike anything you've experienced. The orgasm that results from this kind of stimulation is nonejaculatory, and because you don't ejaculate, there is no recovery period. The stimulation continues to deliver waves of orgasms in a multitude of intensities and lengths, similar to the way a women experiences multiple orgasms.

A prostate-centered orgasm is a powerful, intensely pleasurable event, which, unlike masturbation, shifts you synergistically, connecting body, mind, and spirit. The orgasm might be felt in different parts of your body, such as your prostate (prostate orgasm), rectum and anus (anal orgasm), penis, buttocks, abdomen, legs, or your whole body. Some men have reported multiorgasmic sessions of thirty minutes, while others can go for an hour or longer, resting between waves of intense pleasure.

Partners who have witnessed their lovers in the thralls of this type of orgasmic event report their astonishment at the waves of convulsions and continuous moaning their lovers experience. Photos and videos of men in the throes of these orgasms make it apparent that there's a beginning, middle, and end to these spasms, and as the men are experiencing intense pleasure, the event repeats itself multiple times. Cannabis appears to shift and sensitize the body and mind, while, simultaneously, the prostate massager facilitates or trips the orgasmic wave and intense sexual pleasure.

Additionally, there doesn't seem to be a ceiling to the intensity of these orgasms. As your body becomes accustomed to the pleasure, it continually seeks the next level of orgasmic experience. Cannabis allows us to have full-bodied, unrestricted orgasms—actively opening us to higher octaves of gratification with each new session.

We know so little about the male multiple orgasm and how it affects the body, mind, and spirit, but there is a general consensus among experiencers of a sacrament-infused sexual session that it's a very special and deeply personal event. The Aneros Wiki lists the following as a description for this type of orgasm as "pleasure [that] typically feels bigger, warmer, sweeter, and more encompassing than that felt from the penis stimulation. The sense of excitement you feel might remind you of 'first sex' feelings. The pleasure can spread to large parts of the body and can cause the large muscles of the abdomen and limbs to contract and shake. When the pleasure increases men often find themselves vocalizing involuntarily."

THE MASSAGER AND ANAL PENETRATION

A number of men will be reading this chapter and much of the book, and when they realize that they must stick a device up their ass to generate this new type of orgasm, they will immediately feel uncomfortable. It should be noted that a prostate-centered orgasm is completely new and represents a level of sexual evolution that all men should be aware of and, when possible, undertake steps to achieve. The stigma around inserting a device into the anal canal may bring thoughts of uncleanliness or perversion, or it may seem unnatural to many readers. It should be noted here that you can still experience a great deal of arousal and sexual pleasure without the massager, but with this amazing sex aid, you enter transcending states of bliss that few men have encountered.

If you are heterosexual, experiencing this type of pleasure does not mean that you've suddenly changed your sexual orientation. You are what you are—straight, gay, bisexual, transgendered, and so on—and if you have a prostate gland, this sexual experience is your birthright to enjoy. The orgasmic experience achieved by hundreds of men opens us up to a new awareness of our bodies' subtle pleasure zones. There are thousands of men who are not in touch with their bodies, their physicality, and walk through life unaware of what can give them pleasure and joy. This is also a reason that many men suffer from a wide range of health maladies and die earlier than women. If you have chosen to ignore the messages your body is sending you and power through episodes of pain and discomfort, you walk through life desensitized from your body and its surroundings. Men who are not aware of their body's functions lose the opportunities to explore their sexuality in its full glory.

No matter the shape of your body, so long as you are not dealing with a terminal health condition, you should be able to follow the guidelines in this book to achieve waves of orgasms in a single session and repeat similar events until it's your time to leave the planet.

SELECTING AND USING
A PROSTATE MASSAGER

Earlier, I revealed my preference for the Aneros line of prostate massagers, their design features, and their ability to curate multiple orgasms. Aneros is just one of the many companies claiming that their prostate massagers can provide prostate pleasure leading to an orgasm. An internet search will return hundreds of products of different shapes, sizes, and movements. Some vibrate, while others move in a motion that pokes, rubs, or pushes the prostate gland, triggering an orgasm. But as mentioned earlier, most are poorly conceived, uncomfortable, and in some cases dangerous, placing the user at high risk of damaging the prostate gland. This section will explore what to look for in a massager, from the materials they are made from to how they work.

Prostate massagers are adult sex aids made with the explicit purpose of massaging the prostate. They come in various sizes and shapes but typically follow a standard curved-shaft design with a tapered tip to pinpoint the prostate. Although many guys are wary of anal stimulation, in the past few years the male G-spot and full-body prostate orgasms have become conversational subjects. According to the pleasure-product company Healthy and Active Sex, prostate massager sales have increased by 56 percent over the past five years, particularly among straight men over forty-five.

Additionally, some doctors are encouraging men to perform regular prostate massages (either by doing it solo or with a licensed practitioner), claiming they can potentially help alleviate the symptoms of various health issues. While there is not enough research to suggest that prostate orgasms specifically can lower your prostate cancer risk, generally speaking, having more orgasms is good for your prostate health. According to one Australian study, men who had five or more orgasms per week were 34 percent less likely to develop prostate cancer than men who had one orgasm per week or less.

Choosing a massager that's right for you comes down to preference, comfort, and experience. There are thousands of prostate massage devices on the market, but without a basic understanding of what your body will comfortably accept, the selection process can become overwhelming. Oddly, and as a whole, the prostate massager industry is fixated on producing large, bulky, and poorly designed devices that fill the colon and batter the prostate gland. For our purposes, I provide some guidelines below for selecting a prostate massager, and I list a small group of manufacturers in the reference section, but first, there are some important points to consider in regard to accessing your prostate. To get to the prostate gland requires passage through the anal canal, and this is where we begin our selection process. It's time to get personal . . . *really personal.*

FINDING YOUR PROSTATE

To find your prostate, lie on your side in a fetal position with your legs close to your abdomen. Place a small amount of lube on your finger and insert it slowly into your anus. When the length of your finger is inside, just bend it toward your abdomen, and you'll bump into your prostate gland. As you press this small walnut-sized organ, it will feel spongy and smooth. Don't worry if you don't find it on the first try. No two bodies are the same, and it may take a few attempts to find it. Now that you have manually massaged your prostate gland, let's look at how the prostate massager needs to fit you so as to be effective.

HOW TIGHT IS YOUR SPHINCTER?

To get to the prostate gland, the massager must pass into the anus and the colon to successfully reach the prostate. If you've never attempted this before, you can see why a small massager is a good starting point. Ponder the following statements and decide which best describes you:

- I can hardly get my pinky up there without serious lube.
- I can get two fingers in there before I start yelping.
- I have no problem with butt plugs or other devices.

Once you've decided on your comfort level, determine the type of massager that might work for you, remembering that the compounds in cannabis will heighten prostate sensitivity, and the slightest touch will trigger a spasm. This advice goes for experienced users as well. Newbies will be shocked at the product offerings with large heads and parts that are painful to insert. Although the anal canal can stretch to accommodate a large device, massagers with bulky construction are difficult to insert and uncomfortable to use. What's more, massagers that fill the colon like a butt plug may apply too much pressure on the pros-

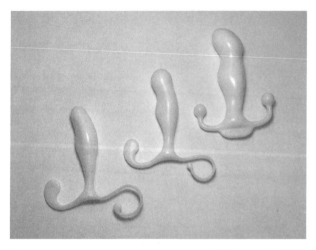

Aneros prostate massagers come in small (Aneros MGX),
medium (Aneros Maximus), and large (Aneros Progasm) sizes.

tate gland and overstimulate it, reducing the likelihood of multiple orgasms. Smaller, simpler massagers are the best solution for a positive outcome.

Once inserted, the device must be hands-free. The head of the massager should rest on the prostate and move freely when you contract your sphincter and pelvic-floor muscles (squeezing and releasing), allowing you to experience the full range of orgasms. When you've had a successful session with multiple orgasms, you can begin to fine-tune which massagers work best for you.

PROSTATE MASSAGER MATERIALS

Prostate massagers come in a variety of different materials. The most sophisticated and versatile are made from silicone, which is the material of choice for those people who enjoy the sensation of a soft and squishy toy. But an equally large population likes a certain rigidity gained from glass, steel, aluminum, plastic, or wood. In either case, look for body-safe materials. These are medical-grade plastics or silicone products. As you get sexually excited, your body temperature will rise, and toys made out of toxic or cheap materials will melt and leak into your insides. Low-quality or cheap toys can result in an allergic reaction, rashes, and other problems you want to avoid.

As you're searching for a prostate massager, you will find hundreds listed on Amazon that look inviting, but buyer beware. Look for reviews on toys you're interested in trying. The best have quality control in their manufacturing facilities and a good review history. Good-to-superior massagers range in price from forty to a hundred dollars.

ELECTRIC VS. NONELECTRIC MASSAGERS

As you discover which massager(s) provides pleasurable stimulation and the eventual orgasm, you'll run across a very large selection of electric massage devices in a variety of sizes and shapes. Although interesting to consider, they're not recommended and not part of the road map to the multiorgasmic man suggested in this book. The electric massager is a mechanical attempt to trigger a prostate orgasm by vibrating or drumming the gland into submission and, with continual use, can damage nerves and surrounding tissue. There are a small number of men who do report great pleasure from using an electric prostate massager, but they risk desensitizing the gland and eventually making it impossible to have a multiorgasmic session.

If you're new to prostate massage, the integration of cannabis and a nonvibrating massager is all that's required to get started. Devices that vibrate or move should be avoided until you can have an orgasm with a nonvibrating massager. Once you've established a routine of multiple orgasm sessions, you're free to experiment with vibrating massagers.

FINAL THOUGHTS ON PROSTATE MASSAGERS

Don't overthink the selection of a massager. Start with a simple-shaped toy. Also note that the more in tune you are with your body and its wellness, the easier it will be to reach high levels of orgasmic pleasure. Eat wholesome foods, reduce your alcohol consumption, stretch, and exercise your body. When you feel good, your body will reward you with exquisite pleasure.

Also remember that a massager should be prostate specific and, for our purposes, used as a secondary stimulant that gently nudges the prostate. The cannabis sacrament is the primary stimulant and launching point for the orgasmic session. While others rely on a massage device alone, adding cannabis is the alchemy that shifts your awareness to a high state of arousal and provides magnificent waves of orgasms.

Once the first waves are delivered and the body is rhythmically processing new orgasms in a period of twenty to thirty minutes, the massager can be removed. At this point the tissues of the prostate have been stimulated enough that the slightest pelvic movements will produce orgasms that are longer and more intense. Eventually, the synaptic connections that lead to a multiorgasmic session will be established, and with proper intent and a relaxed environment the sacrament alone will be all that's needed to have a multiorgasmic session. This is outlined in detail in chapter 8.

As one of thousands of men who for years used a prostate massager without success, I can now state without reservation that the inclusion of the cannabis sacrament and the massager were key components in my rejuvenated sexuality and ability to routinely achieve multiple orgasms at will. The hands-free massager alone is just an instrument on our path to multiple orgasms, and at a point in every man's sexual development, a time will come when the cannabis sacrament alone will be all that's required to achieve similar results. The miracle and the foundation of this book is the sacred sexual sacrament, the compounds in cannabis that set the stage for powerful and repeatable male orgasms, which the prostate massager by itself does not achieve. It's just part of an orchestrated effort that must take place for you to experience a profound sexual event to achieve multiple orgasms.

Keep in mind that this is an entirely new area of sexual experience, so be gentle with yourself. Take your time to experience and encounter your sexual self. If you try to rush through each session, you'll miss the subtle nuances of the experience you intended for yourself.

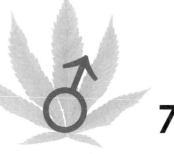

7

The Orgasmic Intention

Manifesting a Multiorgasm Experience

The final step in your journey to becoming multiorgasmic is the process of engaging your unconscious mind and using intention to open your untapped sexuality. In your preparations for a multiple orgasmic event, you've carefully selected a cannabis strain, a prostate massager, and a comfortable environment, and you've given yourself an hour or more of privacy. The last piece of the pre-event activities is setting your intention. Setting an intention unleashes the full range of possible orgasmic outcomes available to you and ensures that the focus of this powerful sexual energy is directed to the prostate as heightened arousal.

When your goal is to have a positive sexual experience, you can increase the chances of that happening by setting an intention. Setting an intention tells your unconscious mind that you want to be open to heightened sexual pleasure and ascend to the highest plateaus of an orgasm. By stating that you intend to have a multiple orgasmic event, you're aligning your mind, body, and spirit to access a full range of possible orgasmic sensations that you may not have previously experienced. In a sense, it's an agreement that allows you to shift into higher octaves of gratification, waves of orgasms that are uniquely your own. The orgasmic intention creates a sexual setting and opens you to an encounter with the most intimate part of your being.

You may be thinking: Why is setting an intention so important? It's just a bunch of words—right? Not exactly. Your sexuality, fully expressed, is the most profound, intimate part of who you are, and when you intend on having an experience that ignites this part of your being, you open to an unobstructed sensual self and engage in the fullest expression of sexual pleasure. Without an intention, your session is left to chance, and the odds are more likely that you will not have the full sexual experience you desire.

From the very first time you start your journey to well into an advanced age, setting an intention for a positive sexual outcome gives your entire being permission to unlock the full range of experiences that grow in intensity and variety each time you engage the prostate. If you've never set an intention, these are key words to consider that will act on your orgasmic outcome. An intention may be as simple as closing your eyes and saying or thinking, "I intend to have multiple orgasms." It might be as sophisticated as saying, "God, Goddess, all that is, I intend to encounter the full range of my sexuality and explore multiple orgasms." Other suggested phrasing is "My intention is to have a powerful multiple-orgasmic experience" or "In this sacred setting, I intend to experience a multiple orgasmic session."

You can also create your own intention by simply stating, "I intend to . . ." then fill in the blank with what it is you'd like to experience. The more creative you are in stating your intention, the better the results. Those who have passed the first phase of achieving repeatable orgasms can consider intentions that broaden the range and intensity of spasms by stating something like, "It is my intention to experience orgasms on multiple levels of consciousness." Here you're opening to very potent contractions that can shift your awareness.

The important part of the intention is the result you want to achieve, and by stating that you intend to have a positive outcome, experience, encounter, event, and so on, you're leaving nothing to chance. You're placing your unconscious mind on notice that you want to have a multiple orgasmic experience.

INTENTION AS GUIDANCE FOR AN ORGASMIC EXPERIENCE

At some point during a multiple orgasmic session, your body may become overstimulated and release control of the experience to your subconscious mind, allowing the autonomic nervous system to take over. In this altered state of consciousness, your brain follows a program, your intention, and leads the body in capturing the stimulus that causes waves of spasms into orgasm. This important point alone is reason to ensure the best possible outcome of your experience by setting an intention.

It's also important to note that during the mind/body/spirit connection, which is induced by the cannabis sacrament, you will never be given more stimulation than you're ready to experience. This is a significant point for individuals who are new to using cannabis and having a prostate-centered orgasm. Depending on the type of strain you're working with and the state of arousal you've achieved, orgasms can range from light waves of pleasure to powerful convulsions that shift your awareness. Cannabis activates a part of our consciousness that works synergistically with the body and opens neural pathways that trigger multiple orgasms. Through our intent, we initiate this process by flagging the prostate gland and marking it to receive stimulation from the prostate massager, and by gently rubbing the prostate, we're telling our brain that this gland is the center of our focus. But here's where it gets interesting. As you encourage an orgasm by massaging the prostate gland, your brain appears to monitor how you respond, and depending on your reaction, will typically increase or decrease the strength and quantity of the orgasms. This may be a protective measure designed into our biology as a safety gauge for these powerful physical reactions to stimulation.

YOUR BEST ORGASMIC OUTCOME

Your intention to have a successful sexual encounter, one that results in multiple orgasms, also engages everything that you've done to make the session as pleasurable as possible. The intention is the glue that adheres the components of your session together and orchestrates waves of orgasmic bliss, which at times, depending on your state of mind and the condition of your body, can reach powerful convulsions. The intention can do the following:

- Direct the cannabis strain to work on opening neural pathways from the prostate to the brain
- Flag the prostate gland as the center of attention
- Provide the sacred sexual setting, ensuring positive results
- Allow you to explore your sexuality within a comfortable environment
- Free you to experience high levels of arousal with a cannabis strain

VISUALIZING YOUR BEST ORGASMIC EXPERIENCE

Another method of creating a successful multiorgasmic experience is to visualize the outcome. It's important to note that the following method is not necessary for a large percentage of men, and stating an intention is usually enough to get the results you desire, but if you have a lot on your mind, are distracted, or feel that you need more to ensure a multiorgasmic experience, adding a visual component can help.

One of the most successful and powerful visualizing techniques is to take a mental snapshot of what you want; for this purpose, an image of you experiencing multiple orgasms. Imagine yourself having a powerful convulsion, an orgasm of great intensity. Then freeze that moment in time. This is the image you will use as you're verbalizing the intention or speaking it in your mind. The combination of a visual image and the verbal intention strengthens the outcome of having multiple orgasms. I would suggest using the visualizing technique each time you initiate a session as you're beginning your journey as a multiorgasmic man. Also, don't be afraid to modify the image before a session and make it as pleasurable as you desire.

A FINAL WORD ABOUT USING INTENTIONS

An intention is your conscious proclamation that you're leaving nothing to chance in your desire for a rewarding encounter with the erotic sexual side of your being. It oversees each portion of the orgasmic experience and conveys your determination to succeed in the process of becoming a multiorgasmic man.

Having multiple orgasms can be exhilarating but also, at times, overwhelming. Having an orgasm that causes tremors or convulsions seems unnatural and counterproductive, but in truth, it's the most natural and healing sexual experience a man can encounter. In this heightened state, we're connecting to the divine and, just for a moment, the ultimate bliss of the human condition.

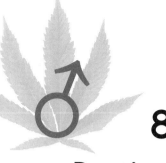

8
Putting It All Together

The Successful Multiple Orgasmic Session

When I discovered that a small dose of cannabis was the key to triggering a multiorgasmic experience, I felt deep gratitude in knowing that my life had been forever changed, and I could initiate a sexual practice that most men only dream about. Note that I used the term *sexual practice* in describing my journey. As much fun as I've experienced exploring this forum of tantric sensuality, I'm extremely respectful of the steps needed to initiate a session and thankful that I've been granted the ability to encounter such profound pleasure.

Now it's your turn.

In its simplest form, this type of sexual pleasure involves a combination of your body, your mind, and your spirit (that other level of consciousness that has been described through the ages as transcended consciousness). Becoming a multiorgasmic man is your birthright, but you must be mindful of this gift and use it in the manner in which it is presented—as a consciousness-expansion tool and a form of sacred sensual invigoration.

There are a number of steps for establishing a lifetime of repeatable experiences and the foundation you'll need to reprogram your brain and nervous system, build arousal, and allow your body to flow with the waves of orgasmic bliss that are generated. The steps outlined in this chapter are based on tried-and-true sessions by many of the men within the Aneros community forum and my own practice. Some of the suggestions may seem time-consuming and distracting, but they are also simple, and each in combination with the others can rewire you to become multiorgasmic in a short period of time. Once you get into a regular practice, you'll find that you're approaching each session with great anticipation and excitement and will no longer see the preparation as work.

THE SACRED SETTING

In the early phase of becoming a multiorgasmic man, choosing a day of the week and location where you have privacy and are not disturbed for a couple of hours sets the stage for a powerful sexually charged event. For those who are new to this experience and as a general guideline, I suggest having sessions of up to two hours two days per week as a goal for rewiring the important synaptic connections needed to have repeatable orgasmic sessions. If you're currently in a relationship and having regular sexual relations in which you have an ejaculatory release, you may require only one session per week. The breaks between sessions are necessary to allow the body a period of rest and recovery and to form the important links for neural plasticity—rewiring of the brain—so you're able to repeat the process.

Though the nervous system is designed to have full-body orgasms, the following are sexual exercises, and in the early stages, they can leave you exhausted as you adjust to the new sensations.

Over time, as you have successful multiorgasmic sessions, you'll begin cementing new pathways from the prostate to your nervous system, brain, and higher guidance. This is a delicate process that takes time, and although you can come out of the gate and try to have a full-blown body-shaking experience every day, if you do not give yourself time to recover, you'll overstimulate the prostate and deaden the delicate nerves and vital connections that must be in place to reproduce multiple orgasms. Give yourself the opportunity to become multiorgasmic throughout your life by allowing a recovery period after each session. I recommend at minimum a full day to rest without stimulation or, for the best results, forty-eight hours between each session to allow your body and brain to regenerate.

For the first ninety days, I recommend choosing two days each week for your sexual practice. These are days when you're able to take an hour or more and place yourself in a quiet and undisturbed relaxed setting. Following is a list of considerations for maximizing your sexual practice:

Choose a day of the week. The goal in becoming multi-orgasmic is the ability to repeat sessions at will and to experience them in sessions that last thirty to sixty minutes or longer. To accomplish this you must choose days when you can completely relax and be mindful of what's taking place while experiencing the sensations your body is producing. To encourage your body, mind, and spirit to deliver what you desire, choose days of the week where you're removed from the pressures of work, family matters, or other distractions. If you're distracted, your mind will not allow you to fully engage, and the experience will not be satisfactory. When you're engaged, you can open to a very high level of arousal, activating your prostate, sexual organs, and your entire body. Choosing the best days and times is a critical starting point to getting the full orgasmic spectrum that is available to you and important for your sexual evolution. If you have a busy schedule, make an appointment each week and add it to your calendar so that you have regular sessions. My practice is Sunday mornings and Wednesday evenings.

Pick an environment. Preparing a space for your practice allows you to open to the experience fully and move through levels of arousal and orgasms. Your bedroom is the ideal location; for most men the bedroom represents a quiet and familiar setting where they can relax fully. Your bed should allow for unrestricted movement and provide the freedom you'll need to stretch and kick your legs and arms freely. If the bedroom isn't appropriate, consider the following:

   a. **The floor.** Throw a large heavy blanket on the floor with a couple of pillows and move furniture and other obstacles out of the way so you have space to move. (Some of my best sessions take place while lying on the floor with complete unrestricted movement.)

   b. **A wide couch.** Although not ideal, adding blankets and a pillow or two to a couch can set the stage for your sexual exploration.

   c. **A motel/hotel.** If you don't have the privacy you need where you live, then consider a local motel or hotel that's in a quiet area. Locations on main streets or busy avenues are not recommended as they will make it difficult to relax and feel comfortable.

Create a sacred setting. Open a window for good airflow, dim the lights, and have a lit candle or two in the room. Your bed or session space should have a couple of pillows, one for your head and one to place between your legs, to allow for a full range of motion. Where possible, stay on top of the bed rather than under the covers to allow your limbs the full range of motion they require. You might even want to remove large comforters or anything that might restrict movement.

Stretch. I highly recommend stretching before a session, with special emphasis on the pelvic region. Important nerves

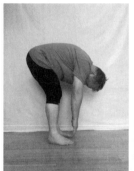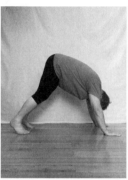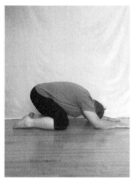

Examples of forward bends.

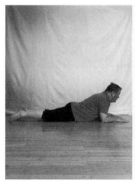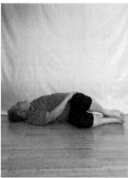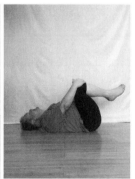

Further examples of how to stretch the pelvis and spine.

connect the prostate to the lumbar region of the spinal column and opening these pathways before your practice can elevate your pleasure significantly. Most of us sit for hours each day, and this has the effect of pinching nerves and cutting off blood flow to the pelvis and our sexual organs. If you practice yoga or any other form of stretching routine, a short twenty-minute program concentrating on the pelvis and abdomen before you start will give you maximum opportunity for a full spectrum of pleasure. If you're not into yoga, a few sustained forward and side bends can help open nerve pathways and increase blood flow to your prostate gland, increasing your arousal and orgasm-response time. Even the simple practice of lying on your back and stretching, twisting your pelvis and spine, can be enough to set a session in motion, unblocking receptors and loosening muscles that will be expanding and contracting. (See sample stretches on page 87.)

Avoid food. A heavy meal before a session is not recommended. If your body is digesting food, it will do two things: send blood and neural input for digestion, taking attention away from your pleasure zones, or stop digestion completely, leaving you feeling bloated. For optimal results, stop eating an hour or more before you engage in a session. If you must eat, make it something light, like a salad, steamed veggies, or egg dishes. Meals with meats are not recommended.

Avoid alcohol. Drinking an alcoholic beverage before a session wreaks havoc on the entire orgasmic process and should be avoided. Alcohol will deaden sensitivity and remove the high levels of arousal needed to trigger multiple orgasms. Also, the effects of alcohol can linger in the system, so it's best to stop drinking at least twenty-four hours before a session.

Drink water. It's important to have a bottle or large glass of water available within easy reach at all times. A variety of cannabis strains tend to dry out the mouth and throat and having some water available relieves this issue. You'll notice that after you've experienced a wave of orgasms, drinking water briefly pulls your awareness out for a moment and refreshes you.

Empty your bowels. Your colon must be empty to enjoy a sexual session, and having a bowel movement is important to maximize the event. If getting a little fecal matter on your massager or hands is an issue, you may also want to use a colonic irrigation device before you begin. If you're dealing with lower bowel, colon, or rectal issues, it's better to wait until the problems have passed before attempting a session. Men faced with hemorrhoids in the anal canal and outside the rectum should be cautious and refer to their health care provider for recommendations. If you've been ill or have a chronic condition, forcing your body to undertake the intense experience suggested here will not provide you with a positive outcome. Also, cannabis has the ability to suspend aches and pains and has a numbing effect on a number of muscle groups. If you've been injured, be aware that the level of orgasms outline in this book can produce strong convulsions and exacerbate a condition.

Wash your body. Shower or bathe, thoroughly cleaning your genitals and anus with a washcloth. Nothing is more invigorating than a hot shower before you enjoy an erotic romp.

This will also help you get in the mood, feeling refreshed in anticipation of sex.

Lubricate. The lubricant you choose is especially important to a positive session outcome. Both the rectum and the massager should be well lubricated so that the device glides over your prostate with the slightest muscle contractions. Before you start a session, you must gently lubricate your rectum and anal canal and apply a thin coat of product to the massager. Aneros recommends ID Glide, which is said to provide sustained lubrication without breakdown, but you may find a product that works better for your needs. If you're unfamiliar with lubricants, your fallback consideration is petroleum jelly, but for maximum massager mobility you will want a water- or oil-based product. You may find that your body reacts to a silicone-based lube with skin rashes and other negative conditions. If you're sensitive to artificial lubricants, consider products that have natural or organic ingredients.

Care for your massager. Once you've selected a device that you feel will work for you, wash it with soap and water before beginning a session and place it within reach.

Set your intention. Setting an intention for the experience you're about to encounter is an important step to ensure that you have a positive multiorgasmic event. Call it whatever you want—a prayer, a call to action, asking for help or guidance—this puts your consciousness, your higher self, on notice that you want a positive outcome during the activity you're about to engage in. See chapter 7 for more details.

Consider using a recording device. In chapter 9, I recommend using a recording app on your phone or an inexpensive recording device that you can place close by to chronicle your sexual practice and your response to the sacrament and massager. This activity is paramount to your reproducing multiple orgasmic sessions.

AN EXAMPLE OF
A MULTIORGASMIC SESSION

To get you started, here's an example of how a session can take shape and lead to a multiorgasmic experience.

The day has come for you to start your practice. The environment is arranged, and you have a couple of undisturbed hours to yourself. Position your massager, lubricant, water, recording device, pillows, and blanket for easy access during the session, then do the following:

- Have a bowel movement or clean your colon with a colonic irrigation.
- Take a hot shower, thoroughly washing with a washcloth.
- In loose-fitting clothing or completely naked, begin your stretching routine, paying special attention to forward bends and other exercises that open the pelvis region of the spine.
- Inhale and exhale deeply as you stretch to oxygenate the blood.
- Set your intention for the session. If this is your first time, ask for guidance as you undertake this journey as well as for a positive outcome. If you're into ceremony (the sacred setting), light a candle as you're setting the intention.
- Get naked (you can keep a T-shirt on if it's cold).

- If you're recording the session, turn on the recorder and log the date and the cannabis strain and massage device you are using.
- Take a small dose of the cannabis sacrament and keep the dispenser (joint, vaper, tincture, etc.) close by for additional doses as needed.
- Lubricate your massager, and place it within easy reach.
- With your fingers, gently lubricate your anus and anal canal.
- Lie down and allow the sacrament to begin shifting your awareness.
- If it's cold, cover yourself with a blanket but still allow for unrestricted movement.
- Visualize the sacrament going to your prostate gland.
- With the massager in hand, slowly insert the device into your rectum.
- Relax and choose a position (on your side, back, or stomach) and feel the massager contacting your prostate.
- Practice a few Kegel exercises, squeezing the sphincter muscle and then relaxing it, directing the attention to your pelvis.
- Close your eyes and visualize your prostate. Breathe in deeply, hold at the top of the breath, and slowly exhale.
- As the sacrament opens you up to the sensations, move your pelvis and sense the massager contacting your prostate.
- As you begin to experience waves of orgasms, allow your body to take over the experience.
- If you're new to prostate massage, you can keep the massager in for the entire session. If you are an experienced user, consider removing the massager at the fifteen- or thirty-minute mark to experience the higher octaves of orgasms.

Prostate orgasms come in all shapes and sizes, and when you begin you may experience slight tickling sensations that roll into pleasurable waves. These will eventually erupt into orgasms, but if they don't, continue to enjoy the ride, staying focused on feeling your prostate. Everyone is different, and for some men, it may take a few sessions to set up nerve pathways that will trigger an orgasmic response. Stay focused on enjoying the session, touching your penis, nipples, chest, and legs as you allow the sacrament to open you up to pleasure. Also remember that having orgasms is just part of the ride, and the heightened awareness of your body is an opportunity to discover your sensuous self by massaging and caressing a variety of awakened erogenous zones. Many men have reported experiencing anal orgasms, nipple orgasms, or, as they get closer to the end of a session and there's a sense the sacrament is wearing off, finishing with a powerful masturbatory ejaculation that in some cases seems to last several minutes.

Keeping your eyes closed can help you connect with the sensations you're experiencing and allow your body to take over the actions. Using a sacrament to release the mind to the unconscious actions of the body signals the beginnings of the ideal sexual union with the body, mind, and spirit. Your body wants to feel the sensations and will move to capture the wave action of orgasms. As the first series of waves pass over you, keep your eyes closed and release control as much as you can. This will allow your unconscious mind to direct the body in whatever moves and positions it requires to capture upcoming stimulation.

Don't get frustrated or feel you've failed if you don't have an earth-shattering orgasm the first time you try. This will only impede your ability to lay new nerve pathways that open you to your sexuality and connect the prostate to the brain (the master sex organ). If you're new to anal play, and inserting a massager into your rectum is a first-time event, this alone may be strange enough to cause momentary alarm. For heterosexual men, fears of change in sexual preference may come to mind. You must suspend this anxiety and look at your sexual practice as an awakening of your God-given sensuality, your ability to develop and experience multiple orgasms. This is where the sacrament can help ease your fears and doubts. Know that in a short period of time, you can repeat your sexual practice and continue to open yourself to the new sensations.

THE STAGES OF A PROSTATE ORGASM

A male G-spot orgasm is triggered by massaging the prostate gland internally, encountering the sensations of the orgasmic wave, riding it to completion, resting, then moving the pelvis or squeezing your anal sphincter just enough to prompt another spasm. Generally, the intensity of these orgasms tends to overwhelm the senses, and as an orgasm surges, passing over the body, most men can do little more than lie back and enjoy the experience. These waves happen in stages and are unique to each person. As you begin to experiment with different arousal strains and prostate massagers and can experience regular orgasms, the following four stages of a cannabis-induced prostate orgasm will become evident:

1. **Altered senses.** The cannabis opens your awareness, and as the intention begins to unfold, you become aware of your body, your genitals, and your prostate. As you focus on this master sex gland, relax into the sensations.

2. **Prostate stimulation.** As you move your prostate massager into place, adjusting it with your anal sphincter muscle and pelvis, squeeze and release your rectum a few times to push and rub the gland.

3. **Trigger point.** As you breathe, the slightest movement of your body pushes the massager against the prostate.

4. **Orgasm.** As the massager connects with your prostate, you'll encounter a powerful orgasm, forcing your body to contract or spasm. These orgasms create a P-wave that radiates outward from the lower abdomen, causing you to feel spacey as it shifts your conscious awareness. After you've experienced a prostate orgasm, you can easily trigger another, although most are involuntary, and the simple act of moving is enough to generate a spasm. As long as a high level of arousal is maintained, some men can keep this orgasmic cycling going for an hour or longer. At some point, there are diminishing returns, and your body becomes exhausted and needs to rest.

Depending on your age and level of health, you can trigger waves of orgasms for an unbelievably long period of time, but there is a point where your body will fatigue, and this is when you should end the session. It's important to remember that a cannabis-induced multiorgasmic event is driven by an artificially induced state of arousal. Although you're in a prone and relaxed position, in a sense you're exercising. As it shifts you sexually, cannabis elevates your heart rate and sensitizes your entire body, mind, and spirit. When you have stopped having orgasms, it's time to rest and revel in the experience you just encountered. Thank the Almighty or your higher guidance and congratulate yourself. You've just entered a new level of human awareness. Yes, you've evolved.

BECOMING OVERWHELMED BY THE SENSATIONS AND STOPPING A MULTIPLE ORGASMIC SESSION

Prostate orgasms are uniquely different from ejaculatory orgasms because they're like an ocean of constant sensation, rising and lowering in waves of intensity as they connect you to your body, mind, and higher levels of consciousness. I've revealed that men are wired to enjoy the pleasures of multiple orgasms, and yet for many first-timers, the intensity can become overwhelming and it's not uncommon for some to experience fear.

Here is where your intention must be employed to set the stage for the experience you will encounter as you initiate a sexual session. When you set an intention to explore the depths of your sexuality in a safe and nurturing environment and to have your guidance watch over the proceedings to ensure the best outcome, your sessions will be powerful and, in most cases, easier to manage. However, it should be noted that a cannabis sacrament can suspend time, greatly amplify your arousal, and open you to levels of sensuality that you've never experienced and may not be prepared to encounter.

In sessions where you're feeling overwhelmed, stop, sit up, take in a few deep breaths, and consume some water. Rejoice in what you're experiencing and thank your guidance, knowing that you've set the stage for a future of sexual pleasure. The new sensations may be scary at first, but as you relax into each wave of orgasm, your confidence will grow and you'll allow yourself to enjoy each level of this new awareness to its fullest.

If, on the other hand, the orgasms become too intense, or you want to stop the session, there are a number of actions you can take that will end a session:

- **Take out the massager.** A good first step to stopping orgasms is to gently take out the massager. Although this may not stop the overall sensitivity that has been activated by the sacrament, it will end the direct contact with the prostate that triggers the flow of orgasmic responses.

- **Stand up.** If you decide to end a session, or you need a break, gently take out your massager and stand up or move to a vertical position on your knees. When you stand, gravity shifts in the pelvis, and the brain changes its awareness from arousal to balance considerations. This will end the sensations. Once you've recovered, you can either end the session or return to a starting position on your side or back and restart the arousal with the massager. Your body will respond in a similar manner if you need to rise to use the bathroom. This on and off technique is good for men who are having trouble managing the intensity of their orgasms and need a breather.

- **Eat something.** When you rise, you will temporarily stop the sensations, but if you have something to eat, you will end the session. The heavier the meal, like having some cold cuts or a meat dish, the faster you'll end the sensations. When you begin eating, the body's dynamics are changed, and its attention goes to digesting a meal. Hot food is also a way to stop most of the arousal you're experiencing.

- **Exercise.** When you stand you temporarily stop the sensations, but if you go further and become physically active by walking, lifting weights, or starting a stretching routine, you will stop the flow of orgasms from the prostate, and as you continue you will end the session.

SOME FINAL THOUGHTS ON PROSTATE MASSAGE SESSIONS

In the beginning of your sexual journey, it's best that you do not have expectations of what you're about to experience. Every man is different, and there are hundreds of factors that come into play when you open yourself to this new sexual awareness. Approaching a session with openness and excitement allows you the space to experience a new form of intimate pleasure and provides time to adjust to the flow of sensations you have never encountered.

I know that there may be other considerations that can be conflicting. For some men, raised in fundamentalist Christian or religious settings, the idea of touching their rectum or inserting a massager may be more then they can comfortably consider. For others who have been shamed as a child to not touch their genitals or rectum other than to urinate or defecate, the idea of a prostate orgasm will not be an option. If you are one of these men, understand that your sexuality is part of being human and prostate massage is an activity that is your birthright to enjoy. This deeply private experience is designed to open you to a new part of yourself, one that allows you to connect with a higher wisdom that the great sages of the past described as Nirvana, or in religious terms, heaven. In fact, having multiple orgasms is one of the most sacred acts you can ever perform as it has the ability to open you to new levels of consciousness and awareness of your time on Earth.

If you can suspend your doubt for just a few hours during a sexual session, the rewards will be life-changing and help you connect with the most intimate part of your being. I'm convinced that this form of sexual awakening is part of an evolution that men around the world can enjoy, and in the midst of their discovery, they can open to a new perspective on their lives. The choice is yours to make: experience profound evolution or remain in sexual stasis.

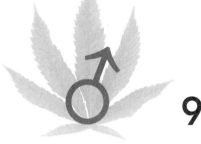

9

Keys to Lasting Sexual Fulfillment

How to Nurture and Retain the Multiorgasmic Encounter

With care, your body can provide you with repeatable multiorgasmic sessions throughout your adult life. As you maintain average-to-good health, and be careful to not overstimulate or injure the prostate, you can duplicate powerful orgasms on a regular basis. I mention average-to-good health because chronic or severe health issues can interfere with the subtle connection between the brain, prostate, and the orgasmic process. More research is needed on this topic, and how the chemicals THC and CBD in cannabis open sensory receptors in the prostate, but ultimately your health is important to having repeatable multiorgasmic sessions.

In this chapter you'll discover how to open yourself to progressively stronger multiorgasmic sessions that are repeatable. I believe this is a new phase in male sexuality, and by having positive multiorgasmic sessions you will open pathways to a source of wellness and higher guidance that you may not have experienced in the past. There is something sacred about this type of orgasmic experience that may have been lying dormant in our physiology until this time in our evolution. It's my belief that having multiorgasmic experiences, and the ability to repeat these sessions with progressively stronger orgasms, opens you to higher levels of consciousness, health, and healing. This connectivity, a communing with the highest levels of our existence, forms a divine connection with the unseen wisdom that guides much of our life. This wisdom or guidance is often called the "higher self."

To achieve repeatable orgasmic sessions and potentially a connection to your higher self, it's important in the early phase of your practice to impress upon the mind, the body, and the higher levels of consciousness an imprint of the experience by means of audio or visual recordings, so that future sessions are easily repeatable. This imprinting phase ensures that your conscious mind becomes aware of your orgasmic experience and locks into memory your self-pleasuring potential.

There's something surreal about this level of pleasure that stretches beyond our everyday experience. Prostate orgasms transcend normal consciousness and can overwhelm you with the intense pleasure your body is receiving, sending you into altered states of awareness. As beautiful as this experience is, there is also an issue of memory retention. Between sessions, you may find that you're actually questioning the experience, wondering if you actually had multiple orgasms or just made up the entire event. As I was discovering my prostate and the pleasure it could provide, there were days when I wondered if I was just lucky to experience one of these rare events. I remember asking myself after a few multiorgasmic sessions if this was real or if the cannabis had influenced the experience to such a degree that my mind, in its altered state, had conjured the entire event, and what I thought were multiple orgasms were actually just an overreaction to the THC and CBD properties within the plant.

Imprinting helps ground the experience in your waking mind, preparing you for future multiorgasmic sessions. Once you repeat pleasurable sessions, the imprinting process can gradually be reduced to the occasional event, although I don't recommend eliminating the process entirely as reviewing sessions helps maintain the status quo of repeatable sessions.

Of even greater importance is the fact that as you climb into higher, altered states of orgasmic bliss, you're connecting with the oldest part of your being and the purest form of consciousness. There may be an occasion where you want to ask a question of your higher guidance and make note of the information that is coming through. The easiest way to do this is to record these events to review after the session. Tools and techniques for doing so are described in the following sections.

RECORDING SESSIONS

Having an orgasm alters our consciousness and opens us up to the exploration of higher states of awareness. Add to this a cannabis sacrament-infused session and you have the makings of a rare and truly remarkable setting where you're linked to your higher guidance in a manner that allows you to become a channel. Wonderful and important information can come through that can benefit you for years to come, so I suggest that you record the sessions. Obviously, this is completely optional, but you'll be amazed at the flow of information you receive that you can listen to in a future setting. As orgasms roll through your body, it's very difficult to remember specific details of what has actually taken place, and impressing on the mind what occurred is important.

Powerful cannabis-induced orgasms can naturally open you to out-of-body experiences in which a part of you resides on higher plains of existence. As you begin to experience multiple orgasms, the intense sensations can overwhelm the brain and send us outside our normal consciousness and into a fog. The ability to repeat orgasmic sessions is a natural extension of the experience, with a caveat: *the goal is to grow each session in intensity* so that we're continually expanding our awareness of higher levels of consciousness and sexual pleasure. Stamping the session with a memory tag (a placeholder) can help cultivate higher realms of orgasmic bliss. Without the memory stamp, you will plateau and possibly simply repeat the previous level of orgasm.

To create the memory stamp, it's important that you duplicate each session in all its majesty and record it to memory. You do this by listening to and/or viewing the immense pleasure you've experienced and realizing that this actually happened to you. Also, as mentioned above, a cannabis-induced session not only sensitizes your awareness of your body, but it also connects you directly to your higher wisdom or guidance (higher self) and can give you a link to access this part of you through question-and-answer and streams-of-consciousness communication.

SETTING THE STAGE
FOR AN AUDIO RECORDING

The simplest method of recording a session is with a handheld recorder. It's important not to interfere with the body's mobility, and for this reason I suggest using the smallest recorder you can find. The ideal recorders are the tiny digital handheld units designed to fit in the palm of your hand. My preference, and the simplest method of recording, is a smartphone. Download your favorite app, and you're ready to go in minutes. I use the Voice Recorder Pro for its simplicity. It's a free app and quickly downloads to your phone. The controls are intuitive, and in short order you can record a session. Don't overthink this and go out and purchase an expensive recording device with special microphones and other hardware. The simple inexpensive recorders are the best.

The recording device should be placed close to your head in a location that does not hinder your ability to move as needed. I've found that when lying in bed, placing the recorder at the top of my headboard or at the head of the mattress, closest to the headboard or at the farthest corners of the mattress, but not so far that any movement would shake it off the bed, is a good location. Before you start your first session, practice by placing the recorder in a few different locations and recording yourself talking, breathing, coughing, and so on. When you play back this test, you should be able to hear yourself clearly so that at the end of a session and experience you'll realize what has happened.

Additional Tips

After you have placed the recorder in the ideal location, turn on the mic and forget it. At the start of your session, proceed in the following manner:

- Record the date and time of the session.
- Describe how you are feeling as the sacrament is beginning to take effect.
- Express the first thoughts that are coming to mind as the sensations are passing through you.
- Ask a question or two to see if an answer comes forth.
- Release mental control and allow the body to take over and proceed with the session.

As the sacrament takes effect, your body will begin to move in anticipation of approaching orgasms, leaving you to ride along with the experience, and as you pass through this multiorgasmic bliss, the recorder will pick up both your subtle and unrestrained outbursts and provide you an opportunity to replay the session. Don't be afraid to continually move the recorder around the bed (maintaining close proximity to your head) as you're having an orgasm. After the session, listening to your convulsions, breathing, and movements is a joyous experience that will make you laugh, cry, and revel in the realization that you're a multiorgasmic being. You will be amazed at what you're hearing and giggle and laugh along with that person (yes, that's you) passing through orgasmic waves of pleasure.

By recording your sessions, you capture and reinforce the experience in your memory. This memory will help you to repeat these sessions in the future, open to increasingly stronger and more multiexperiential orgasms, and pave a path to begin working with your higher guidance. Audio recordings are one of the foundations of your lifelong journey of exploring and maintaining a multiorgasmic awareness.

VIDEO RECORDING SESSIONS
(OPTIONAL)

Another method for retaining sessions is video recording. Observing yourself in a session is educational, fun to watch, and represents one of the most sacred sexual experiences you'll have in your lifetime. Here again, the act of watching reinforces the multiorgasmic experience so that it's repeatable.

I've made this optional only because videotaping isn't for everyone and may require a significant financial output. But if you're a visual learner, watching yourself may be the best avenue to reinforce your experiences so that they're easily repeatable. If you search the web for prostate orgasms, you'll discover a small number of video sessions conducted by men of all ages. If you're a heterosexual man, you may find watching nude men a little uncomfortable, but once you move past this, these videos can be educational if not a little erotic. As a heterosexual man, I've found that watching others pass through the bliss of a multiorgasmic session is both fascinating and educational. Most, if not all, are lost in the moment as they thrash about on beds, sofas, and other settings. Take note of what prostate massager is being used, as well as the resting positions and the convulsive orgasms these men are experiencing. It's interesting to note that no two men are alike and each presents a unique rite of passage. Although it's not known if any of the men in these videos used the cannabis sacrament in their sessions, each provides a look into how a multi-orgasmic session affects individuals differently.

Capturing your orgasmic events on video allows you to review your sessions in all their glory, and studying yourself and the variety of orgasms passing through you reinforces the event and marks your arrival into a new evolved you.

Equipment and Setting Basics

This is one of the most sacred and personal experiences you will ever have in your life, and you may prefer to be alone while you're having it. On the other hand, it's also the pinnacle of sexual bliss, so you may want to include a lover to join you as you're moving through orgasms. There is no right or wrong way to pass through these events, and how you experience a session is completely up to you. However, as I mentioned, it's my belief that this type of sexual experience is designed to connect you with your higher guidance and provide you an opportunity to understand your purpose in this lifetime as well as vital information on your path. And if you're interacting with another person, the information that comes to you during an orgasm, either through questions and answers or just blurting out statements, may be missed. It's for this reason that I strongly urge you to begin your journey on your own and discover how your body reacts to the new stimulation.

In terms of equipment, again, less is more and getting a basic video camera and tripod should not break the bank. Also, depending on the space you're using, you might need a couple of lights to ensure that you're well lit for the recording.

I'm not going to go into what equipment to buy or the best brands for the occasion in this book. There are a multitude of camera options from which you can select, and given the high quality of even the least expensive brands, you'll be able to get the best equipment for your needs. This is also true for tripods, although I've found that tripods made of steel rather than plastic are a better choice for stability. Here again, the decision is ultimately yours to make. Just remember that your goal is to capture your orgasmic adventure as simply and as clearly as possible.

I will advise you, however, to purchase a memory card that is sixty-four gigabytes or larger so that you can capture an entire session. I recommend the SanDisk card for videos. Under normal settings, this will record for two-plus hours or more and will provide a recording that you can upload to your computer.

Before and After a Session

Before your session, attach the camera to the tripod and position it so that it's elevated above your bed. Some might like the camera placed at the foot of the bed, while others may prefer the side. Get a wide-angle shot that covers the entire mattress. Remember that you'll be thrashing about, and you'll miss the details if you focus down too tightly. Turn on the camera and record yourself in a test run to see how you look. Roll on your back, stomach, and sides as you normally would when sleeping. Play back these tests to see if you've captured the important details. Check the volume control and adjust as needed following your tests. Once the image and sound are balanced you're ready to record.

Following the session, save the recording so you can watch it privately. Observe how you reacted to the sacrament and note what took place. Keep a journal of your sessions and note the following:

- Name of the sacrament cannabis strain you were using
- Dose (one or more draws or puffs) of the cannabis strain
- How you felt when you used it
- Brand and model of the prostate massager
- Length of your session
- Strength and types of orgasms
- Comments

Keep it simple, with short paragraphs. These notes will assist in reinforcing the experience.

STAYING IN GOOD PHYSICAL SHAPE (SEXERCISES)

No one wants to have sex when they're feeling ill, low on energy, or depressed. Your body should be the center of your universe, the tool that can provide you with the ultimate physical experience—powerful, repeatable orgasms. My guess is that just about any boy or man of average sexual maturity can have multiple orgasms, and as soon as you can experience an ejaculation and your prostate is functioning properly, your body will be ready to handle a multiorgasmic session.

When men are young, having an ejaculatory orgasm is a regular event. Masturbating is something all of us do when our hormones are raging and we're discovering our bodies. This is a normal and healthy practice. Now, by using the techniques outlined in this book, every boy or man has the opportunity to experience multiple orgasms, whenever or wherever they choose, with one slight caveat: you must be in a state of wellness that allows your body to receive the sensory input that takes place between your prostate, brain, and higher guidance.

You don't have to be a gym rat to become a multiorgasmic man, but it's important to stay in good-to-average shape, so your body can fully experience the sensory pleasure of a session. I believe that the physical experience of multiple orgasms is natural and that all men can enjoy the experience on a regular basis. But because many of us work for hours at a time in environments that are sedentary, have not been encouraged to enjoy the outdoors, or live in climates that discourage regular physical activities, we don't take care of our bodies. If you do not take pride in your body and work to stay well, you will not experience the part of your being that is multiorgasmic. You don't have to look like a movie actor or ripped weight lifter, but it's important to be well and feel good. And you must have good blood flow to your organs, especially your prostate gland. This requires that you exercise, or sexercise, paying particular attention to stretching. Exercises that raise the heart rate and stretch the body are the best tools to prime the orgasmic pump.

However you choose to sexercise, *avoid your phone!* I love my smartphone and take it with me wherever I go. It's become a part of my existence, but it's also a bit addicting and can intrude on my daily activities. Make it a standing rule that when you sexercise, you leave the phone in your pocket, in the car, or at the house. DO NOT, I repeat DO NOT have it available when you sexercise. You must relieve your body, mind, and spirit of the noise and unwanted stimulation that your phone provides. You defeat the purpose of the sexercise when you take your phone with you.

You must create a routine where you are getting regular sexercise to maintain the health and responsiveness of your body. Following are a few suggestions for exercises that will support a growing orgasmic awareness.

Yoga

Stretching is a key component in experiencing the higher orgasmic levels that will rock your body, and yoga is the ultimate sexercise that will prepare your body, mind, and spirit for the multiorgasmic experience. It's also one of the main factors in cultivating powerful orgasms that can give you extreme pleasure. When I think of my yoga practice, which I do three days per week, and how it seamlessly interconnects with my sexual practice, it's as though the two were designed for each other. Yoga opens and concentrates on portions of the body that are vital to triggering the flow of orgasms while massaging the organs and relieving the practitioner of accumulated toxins and stress that can reduce the orgasmic experience. I suggest a short twenty-minute yoga session to open pathways before you retire to your sacred space and begin a session.

You might also consider attending a weekly class with a trained yoga teacher. After you've discovered a series of positions that work for you, you can create a practice at home. Yoga was designed for all ages and health conditions and when practiced routinely will help you to maintain optimal wellness and experience the higher levels of intense orgasms well into an advanced age. Your yoga routine should have equal parts of stretching the upper and lower body, paying special attention to the pelvis and lower back. An open and flexible pelvis is the key to good prostate health and a multiorgasmic body (see p. 87).

Walking and Hiking

Walking is one of the best methods of getting the exercise your body requires for sexual fitness. A twenty- or thirty-minute walk outside a few days a week will raise your heartbeat enough to maintain good body functions, clear the mind of the day's activities, and flush your system of toxins and other metabolic issues that can stagnate good elimination. Moving your body also increases your sexuality and sexual awareness and opens new pathways for engaging with your world more optimistically.

I live close to a regional park and find that light hikes (no more than an hour) are ideal for clearing my mind and providing the prerequisite cardio exercise needed for maintaining good health. There's also something about getting off the pavement or cement that's rejuvenating. It's a signal, perhaps an unconscious one, that I'm in nature and allows for absorption of the raw elements.

I believe that one of the biggest issues surrounding wellness is the fact that we've forgotten to connect with nature and that living in an environment void of greenery and other natural elements can cause us stress and illness. Getting outside and into a natural setting assists the body in maintaining an equilibrium that will help in developing your sexual awareness. You may find that getting out for a brisk hike is something that you'll look forward to, and when you return home, you've cleared the distractions and can move into the next phase of your day or evening with renewed energy and purpose. I can't say enough about day hikes. I take them two to three times a week to maintain wellness. Together with my yoga practice, I have plenty of sexercise to support my orgasmic practice.

Biking

Cycling on a stationary or regular bike is a great way to exercise. Most of my friends who are bikers are slim and trim and have an optimistic outlook on life. If you've ever considered taking up bike riding, do so. Over time, it can provide you with great coordination, and combined with a stretching routine, it can optimize your multiorgasmic sessions.

A note about inside vs. outside exercising: Not all of us live in climates that are optimal for year-round outdoor exercise. It may be too hot or too cold where you live to get outside for an exercise routine every day, but whenever possible, you should be out in the fresh air, moving your body. We need sunlight to maintain good health, so even when it's not ideal, go outside and move around a couple days a week.

Other Exercises

I've listed just a few exercise suggestions that can optimize your wellness and sexual vitality. Remember that incorporating a stretching routine into your weekly exercise program a couple of days a week is important for experiencing the higher level, intense orgasms that transcend a regular experience. There are many other exercises—such as weightlifting, running, swimming, and martial arts—that you can do to increase the blood flow to your organs and the prostate gland.

YOUR EMOTIONAL WELL-BEING AND ORGASMS

An open and positive mental/emotional state of mind are a prerequisite for the multiorgasmic man. You should be excited about the journey you're about to start and anticipate each new session with optimism and joy. I've found that as I'm getting close to my session day, my body, mind, and spirit are fully engaged and tingling. It's this knowing what's about to come that's exhilarating. After each completed session, you'll discover a deep satisfaction that you've experienced a truly transcendent event that only you can reproduce. But many of us are struggling with the weight of our lives and have a less-than-positive outlook.

Depression is rampant in our society, and a large number of prescription drugs are dispensed each year to combat this problem. Exercise has been proven to reduce depression and a host of other emotional problems we encounter in our lifetime. If you're sad, depressed, or unhappy, this will impede your multi-orgasmic sessions and lessen your ability to enjoy your sexuality. Using the cannabis sacrament may be a way to improve your emotions in a positive manner, but this should be taken with a caution.

There are mixed reviews on using cannabis for depression, and in some clinical studies serious complications were noted. Some studies reported that cannabis can make the person struggling with this affliction worse or lead to other serious psychological issues. But a growing number of studies show that for short periods of time, cannabis may suspend depression and allow for a more optimistic outlook.

Because of the powerful medicines in antidepressant drugs and their effect on the brain and nervous system, if you are taking antidepressants I would advise against consuming the cannabis sacrament, as this could cause adverse effects and unwanted reactions. If you already combine the two, then remember to use the sacrament in small doses. It's important to consult with your health care provider to determine how you will metabolize the sacrament.

Obviously more research on the effect of cannabis on depression and other emotional states is needed, but it's my belief that as you experience a multiple orgasmic session, you will find yourself more optimistic and positive about your life and those around you. The combination of the prostate massager and the relaxed setting may be enough to trigger the explosive orgasms.

Obviously if you're emotionally upset, stressed, or worried about something, you're not going to be in the mood for a sexual experience. To limit this, I suggest choosing a day when you will not be bothered by outside distractions and are free for a couple of hours of privacy.

SACRED SETTING

There are a few lifestyle changes that must be considered if you want to experience the full spectrum of prostate orgasms. The higher octaves of this ecstasy are available only to those who can control their environment and maintain a balance of work and play. Following are some suggestions for doing so:

Get enough sleep. You must have sufficient sleep to maintain good body awareness. Everyone has different sleep needs, but as a rule, most of us need seven hours of solid rest. More is great, less can become problematic. If you're chronically exhausted, you have few reserves left to experience your full potential of an orgasmic man. A well-rested body translates to powerful orgasmic sessions. Adjust your schedule so that you get to bed on time and develop good and repeatable sleep patterns. Once you've created a bedtime routine, you'll look forward to completing the activities of the day and moving into the important sleeping time. I've always had a bad habit of staying up into the early morning hours, then waking up to my alarm, groggy and, at times, exhausted. I recently discovered that my phone has a sleep mode built into the clock app that I can set to get my seven hours of sleep. It subtly and gently reminds me to go to bed at 12:30 a.m. by playing a few musical notes from Brahms's "Lullaby." It then plays my choice of music at 7:30 a.m., and I wake feeling refreshed. If your job or current life situation demands a good deal of your attention, or your daily stress levels are high, you may require more sleep. Setting the app for more or less sleep time is a simple adjustment.

Avoid alcohol consumption. I love beer and wine and on occasion overdo it a bit when sampling some of the amazing craft-style beers that have emerged on the scene where I live. As good as it tastes, alcohol reduces or impedes important synapse connections in the brain and greatly reduces the sensations of the prostate gland. Never drink an alcoholic beverage before a session; in fact, avoid all alcohol on the day you've designated for a session. (For more information on alcohol consumption, go to "The Sacred Setting" in chapter 8.)

Limit sessions to cultivate powerful orgasms. For the vast majority of men, a multiorgasmic session will be unlike any sexual experience they've encountered before. The nonstop flow of powerful orgasms is an intensely pleasurable sensation that can last for more than an hour, and similar to masturbation, as the body recovers from a session, there may be a desire to repeat the experience again as quickly as possible. However, through my own trial and error and that of the hundreds of men who have reported their experiences, attempting a repeat session immediately after a successful multiorgasmic experience produces poor results. It appears that the prostate needs time to recover. Unlike the penis, which is the center of attention when you masturbate, the prostate sits inside your body and is not surrounded by skin or protective tissue. The gland is hidden behind a thin layer of tissue, the colon wall, which can tear or be damaged by repeated stimulation. Therefore, it's preferable to wait a couple of days or more before repeating a session so that the prostate has time to recover, regenerate, and build new sensory pathways to the nervous system and the brain. For me, limiting sessions to one or at most two times a week produces orgasmic sessions that are the most memorable.

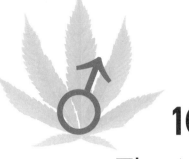

10

The Nonresponsive Session and Other Problem Areas

Solutions and Affirmations for Cultivating a Prostate Orgasm

If you follow the guidelines listed in chapter 8, you should see positive results after your first few attempts. However, it is important to remember that each of us is unique, and we metabolize the chemical compounds in cannabis differently. Some will have sensations that unfold quickly and produce intense feelings of arousal, triggering rapid orgasms, while others may encounter sessions that build gradually, with orgasms that have peaks and valleys.

For some, the rituals laid out in this book may require a short adjustment period that allows for the integration of cannabis and the sensations caused by its use. Newbies may need to get comfortable with the elevated arousal, the prostate massager, and their own sensuality before relaxing into an orgasm. Whatever you experience, be patient and know that future sessions will continue to grow in sensation, strength, and intensity. Cannabis-fueled multiple orgasm encounters involve a collective that syncs your body, mind, and spirit. During a session, your heart rate and body temperature are elevated, and as waves of powerful spasms pass over you, the experience will be similar to a demanding cardio exercise.

It may take a few sessions to get comfortable with a strain that you're unfamiliar with, or you may find yourself too high and must wait to come down before beginning your massage session. Whatever the case may be, it's essential to be patient and let experiences unfold as you relax into them, knowing that they will keep growing and expanding with time. You will eventually get into a rhythm, a methodology that you use before, during, and after each session that reminds you of the path to sexual gratification and multiple orgasms.

TIPS FOR ALLOWING PROSTATE ORGASMS TO HAPPEN

If you don't have an orgasm the first time out, don't despair. Know that your body and higher guidance want you to have the experience you desire, but you may need to make some adjustments first. These adjustments may include one or more of the following:

- Acknowledging that you are a sexual being with wants and desires
- Overcoming fear or a low comfort level with exploring your body and touching your penis, nipples, anus, and so on
- Becoming comfortable with your sexual expressiveness so that you can let go enough to enjoy the pleasure

- Creating a comfortable and quiet space where you can be undisturbed
- Discovering how to consume cannabis to feel consciously altered without becoming too high
- Learning to use a prostate massager and becoming comfortable with the many sensations it can generate
- Feeling safe enough to release into the sensation of arousal, the precursor to an orgasm
- Riding the waves of orgasms that pass over you

Problems with any one of these areas may block you from having the sexual encounter you desire. In addition, you may occasionally feel stuck, unable to move into a positive alliance with yourself. In these situations, consider turning problems into positive affirmations that over a short course of time can change the outcome of your sessions.

Generally speaking, affirmations are used to reprogram the subconscious mind to encourage us to believe certain things about ourselves or about the world and our place within it. They can also be used to help us create the reality we want—often in terms of making (or attracting) wealth, love, beauty, and happiness.

While this concept may sound to you like a load of psychobabble, positive affirmations have been shown to quickly change your perspective, help lighten the emotional load, and shift negatives into positives. Following are a few examples to get you started:

- It's safe for me to explore my sexuality.
- I'm open to receiving the pleasure I desire each day.
- I love and accept my body and the pleasure it provides me.
- Each and every day, I'm becoming a multiorgasmic man.

Of course, cannabis, too, can act as a buffer against issues that may seem insurmountable. When you engage this medicinal plant helper, you open to more profound and gratifying emotional and physical experiences while ushering in the hopes, desires, and, above all, the intentions you've set for a successful outcome. Unlike getting high to chill out, when you actively engage cannabis in a sexual encounter, the plant shifts your awareness and consciously guides you to the ultimate goal—a powerful, full-body prostate orgasm. But you may find yourself in situations where cannabis alone may not be enough to provide you with a sacred setting, one that nurtures your gratification. The next section will help you better understand what may be getting in the way of your pleasure.

OTHER ISSUES THAT CAN HAMPER PROSTATE ORGASMS

There are several other circumstances that can hamper a multi-orgasmic experience. These include personal upbringing and societal pressures, settings and situations, work or personal issues, and health problems. Let's look at each of these problem areas in turn, along with some solutions for overcoming them.

Personal Upbringing and Societal Pressures

Unleashing and enjoying your sexuality is simple enough to consider, and yet for many men, admitting that they're sexual beings brings up feelings of embarrassment, resentment, and shame.

We were all raised in different environments that affected how we view sexuality, self-pleasuring (masturbation), and sexual relations. The connection to our sensuality may have been determined early on by our parents' views on sex, our religious indoctrination, and society's level of acceptance. Many of us were raised to resist the temptation of exploring our sexuality and the multitude of erogenous zones that are part of a man's body. As children we were admonished for touching our penis and rectum or enjoying our sensuality. If you feel uncomfortable exploring your body, it may be due to a number of different factors that occurred in your childhood. For example, if you were shamed when you asked questions about sex or were caught exploring your body and told it was filthy, you may experience feelings of remorse, self-loathing, and guilt that can play a large part in blocking you from having a positive sexual outcome.

Here is where cannabis can serve as a powerful tool to get you unstuck from your past and help move you into a more positive state of mind. Most people enjoy the sensation of being altered consciously that cannabis provides. Feelings of guilt or shame are pushed aside, opening you to the sensations and awareness of your body.

Settings and Situations

To experience the full dimension of your sexual expression and self-pleasuring, you need to have a location that allows you a couple of hours (minimum) where you will be undisturbed. The setting should also be quiet, inviting, and allow you the freedom to stretch out on a couch, bed, or the floor.

If you're in a relationship, explain to your partner the importance of what you're setting out to accomplish. Some men are comfortable with and enjoy including a lover in the process of opening to a new sexual experience. But this isn't a regular romp in bed. As previously discussed, the beginning phase and early exploration of your prostate gland includes rewiring the response reflex, redirecting focus and energy to your prostate, and riding the sensations delivered by the massager. You're telling your mind, body, and spirit that you want a sexual encounter that includes multiple orgasms.

Although the process is fun, any distractions can delay the onset of the orgasm waves, so as suggested earlier, go solo for the first few sessions. Until you can comfortably sense when the effects of the cannabis, the prostate massager, and the other components leading to multiple orgasms have been achieved, you should not have any outside interference. Also, when you're solo, you can express yourself fully by groaning, laughing, convulsing, and crying during a session without feeling inhibited by another's presence.

Work or Personal Issues

We all experience times when work or personal problems weigh heavily on our minds. Work situations and personal relationships have their peaks and valleys and can often cause stress and dissatisfaction. While it may not be best to pursue your sexual desires during times of conflict, if you find that you're in the mood for some sexy play, cannabis can deliver a reprieve from these problems by shifting your awareness to the task at hand—a wonderful full-body orgasm. The great advantage of strains that are designed to elevate your horniness is that once you've started a session, the pleasure continues to grow, and as you're shaking from a convulsive spasm, nothing else matters. These private sessions can free you from the problems of the day—be they caused by family, friends, or work associates—and allow you to engage selfishly in a few hours of sexual abandonment.

Health Problems

Health issues can impede your ability to experience any kind of sexual exploration and body functions that produce an orgasm. Still, the human body is amazingly resilient and, even when it's not at 100 percent, can take you to amazing sexual heights. As a general rule, the better you care for and maintain your health and wellness, the more pleasure you'll experience with the cannabis-infused sexual exploration I've outlined. Consider taking vitamins and prostate supplements to help improve and maintain a healthy prostate and avoid infections and irregularities of this amazing gland. Look to the resource section for websites with tips to maintain a healthy and active prostate gland and heal infections and recommendations for what to do when you receive dire news about your prostate.

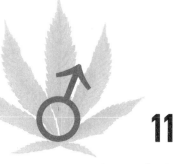

11
Multiple Orgasms, Obsession, and Addiction
Setting Goals for Your Sexual Awakening

The powerful sexual stimulation associated with multiple orgasms will eventually change a man's attitude toward his body and can develop into a life-altering experience—one that runs the risk of becoming an addiction. Because of this possibility, I've found that it's important to treat each experience with a sense of reverence and place it in a sacred setting so that you're mindful of what's taking place as you engage in multiorgasmic pleasure. Without this respect for the process, you can quickly cross the line into sexual addiction.

As I've outlined in this book, the effects of cannabis are not a new discovery. The compounds within the drug have been used for thousands of years as powerful sexual stimulants. Because cannabis links neural pathways and turns up arousal, both men and women who were once incapable of having an orgasm can find cannabis helpful in achieving not one but multiple orgasms. Also, multiple orgasms are just one part of the cannabinoid effect. There are levels of orgasmic intensity that are delivered to the user that can range from full-body convulsions to mind-bending ecstasy that leave one breathless and produce a type of spiritual awakening that most only read about in metaphysical books. I'm here to suggest caution when you approach this form of sexual awakening and to be respectful of your body when you introduce the sacrament. Here is where I urge you, again, to consider that less is more.

As you experiment with microdosing different cannabis strains *with intention,* you'll begin merging higher levels of consciousness and experience profound sexual bliss. However, if you overuse or abuse cannabis on a daily basis or without proper rest, you will eventually lessen the effects of the stimulant, desensitize the prostate, and irreparably damage the gland and your ability to have multiple orgasms.

In addition, a number of medical journals report incidents of "unexpected orgasms" in men and women who use cannabis during sex and climaxes lasting for several minutes at a time. It turns out that THC and CBD in combination are powerful stimulators and, when abused, can cause the user to experience uncontrolled orgasmic responses to the degree that many must seek medical intervention.

The important take away from these incidents is the addictive nature of this sexual experience. Cannabis can thrust you into pleasure zones that will leave you gasping for air and thoroughly exhausted. It suspends time, ramps up arousal, and delivers profound sexual pleasure that will leave you amazed and wanting to experience more as soon as possible. It can be powerfully addictive, and this can become a problem. The next section provides suggestions for ensuring that you do *not* cross the line into problem areas and become addicted to the multiorgasmic experience. In addition to the suggestions given, I would also suggest seeking out men's groups (online or in person) where men can get together and discuss their sexual awakenings and the changes and experiences associated with being multiorgasmic.

SETTING GOALS FOR YOUR SEXUAL AWAKENING

If you can set goals early on your path to becoming multiorgasmic, you're less likely to delve into addictive behaviors that can result in long-term damage to the prostate. Goal setting can also help you avoid traps like repeating sessions too soon or consuming cannabis to such a degree that you must take greater amounts for any effects to be felt or that gets you so high that you completely lose awareness of your practice and move beyond the pleasure zone required for triggering orgasms.

As our understanding of the effectiveness of cannabis continues to grow, the idea of getting stoned must be reconsidered and replaced with a new awareness of the positive effects of the sacrament and its ability to connect the mind, body, and spirit. Setting goals can help you achieve a positive integration of cannabis in your life as you awaken your sexuality. The list below provides several suggested goals to get you started:

- Repeating multiorgasmic sessions
- Discovering the higher octaves of orgasms
- Connecting with your higher self or guidance
- Becoming a better lover

Repeating multiple orgasmic sessions should be paramount for men of all ages and an important consideration for a lifetime of gratifying sexual pleasure. One of the main purposes in writing this book is to make you aware of the high levels of arousal produced by microdoses of cannabis and the different strains you can use to experience multiple orgasms. But the sacrament doesn't stop there, and as you continue to use cannabis in your sessions, you'll discover that having an orgasm can become as easy as breathing deeply and squeezing your sphincter muscle. Eventually the prostate massager will not be required to stimulate an orgasm, and you're able to have them with just the cannabis sacrament. This takes time and can only happen if the prostate has been conditioned early in your practice, and you give your body sufficient time to recover following sessions.

Essentially, the process requires activating, growing, and sensitizing the nerves in the prostate that connect to the spinal column and lead to the brain (your master sex organ.) Early in the process, your body and brain are reliant on the stimulant in cannabis, which has the ability to greatly slow down time and allow the body to experience very high levels of arousal. Once these powerful prostate orgasms have been experienced, the brain and body work to repeat the experience. We're still in the dark as to how this happens and what an orgasm actually does to the body and brain, but it's my belief that the sensations of multiple orgasms are a natural evolution for men, designed to open and shift our awareness to new levels of conscious awareness.

Discovering the higher octaves of orgasms is part of the journey, and exploring the sensations associated with different types of orgasms should be every man's goal once they have established regular and repeatable sessions. As your body becomes more comfortable with each experience, and you allow yourself to enjoy your body, your higher guidance will begin delivering orgasms of greater strength and intensity and in longer duration. I believe these sensations are in direct response to the opening of neural pathways and communing with the higher realms of consciousness that, in general terms, oversee these activities.

By introducing the cannabis sacrament, a number of men have documented multiple orgasms of such great intensity that they were removed from their physical presence and elevated into levels of consciousness that they described as transcendent, or out-of-body, experiences. I've had a few of these, and they're exhilarating and magnificent. These orgasms were manifested through the careful adherence to once-a-week practice, proper stretching, food restrictions, and setting an intention. These transcendent experiences should be the goal of every man's sexual awakening, as they mark an evolutionary leap that appears to have positive long-lasting effects.

It's important to note here that it's highly unlikely that you will achieve these higher level orgasms if you're abusing the process and overstimulating the prostate or repeating sessions without regard for body function. The greater your awareness for the actions taking place when you have multiple orgasms, the better prepared you'll be to receive pleasure at the level of intensity that will leave you breathless and thanking your higher guidance for such a glorious experience.

Connecting to your higher self may be another of your goals for having multiorgasmic experiences. Western science and Judeo-Christian ethics have failed to gain an understanding of what older cultures in India and China term higher levels of consciousness, or the higher self. But in a nutshell, it is the idea that we are multidimensional beings and possess physical, mental, and higher levels of self (or being). Our higher self (sometimes also thought of as the soul) is considered to be the master essence of our being and the driver of our daily awareness and oversees much of what we do and how we go about our daily activities. The more we can connect with this higher self, the more success, wellness, and happiness we can experience in this lifetime. A goal of connecting more thoroughly with our higher self means a life of more fulfillment and pleasurable interactions.

Becoming a better lover should be every man's goal, and as you become a multiorgasmic being, you'll discover that you're a pleasure seeker who wants and needs to experience your orgasms but also help your partner to enjoy their sexual awakening. As a multiorgasmic man, you've entered a very high level of sexuality and have experienced a sexual awakening that most men are not able to achieve. Having multiple orgasms will open you to your sensual self, and connecting with a lover allows for other opportunities to discover sexual arousal on different levels.

This is also a deeply intimate opening to nurture another person and transcends simple sex. When you become a multiorgasmic man, you'll want those you're intimate with to experience the pleasure you experience and will go the extra mile to ensure their satisfaction. Helping another person have an orgasm or multiple orgasms will become your goal, and as a sexual pleasure seeker you will enter the place of becoming a conscious (better) lover. This makes for a great relationship that has more opportunities to thrive in our complicated world.

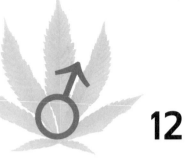

12

Using Cannabis to Express Yourself Sexually

Now It's Your Turn to Experience Bliss

The idea for this book came to me in the fall of 2018, but it wasn't until later that all the pieces came together, and science finally caught up with this sacred weed and clarified a number of important issues. After months of research and personal discovery, I knew I had to write about my experience and share it with others, especially since I was the program director for the San Francisco Cannabis Business Summit at the time. My intimate revelations and those of a growing number of men and women represent a new look at marijuana and how it can dramatically improve intimacy and the sacredness of sex. Perhaps of equal importance was the discovery of the male G-spot (the prostate gland), the addition of a prostate massager, and the resulting multiple orgasms.

For years, I was curious about India's Tantra temples and the motivation for depicting thousands of different couples in coital positions carved on the walls and celebrated for centuries as an homage to Lord Shiva. I now realize the complexity of the cannabis plant and how it could open them to new levels of conscious awareness, the purpose of incarnating physically, and the great pleasure achieved by integrating cannabis with sexual expression. Cannabis was sacred to our ancestors, and soon, we'll revere it again.

Cannabis advocacy is growing worldwide, and here in North America, as more states legalize its recreational use, a broad and enthusiastic audience will discover a new definition of sex—either with a partner or by themselves—and its summation we call orgasm. I can still remember my disbelief when I experienced the magnitude of the spasms brought about by a prostate orgasm for the first time. A few years ago, as a member of the Aneros forum, I knew that a small percentage of men who used a prostate massager were able to trigger this experience, but I had no idea that cannabis could be the key to a multiorgasmic encoun-

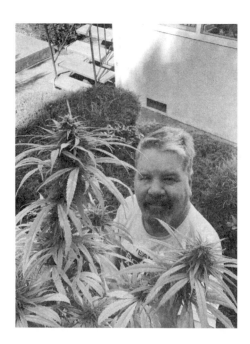

Cannabis is surprisingly easy to grow in most climates. This is Blue Dream, about ten days from harvest.

ter. Cannabis is the game changer that levels the playing field and provides every man and woman immediate and unrestricted access to orgasmic pleasure in a safe and measured setting. This plant medicine is a gift for all of us.

As a suggestion, if you have limited experience with marijuana, consider exploring the sensations different strains can produce before undertaking the steps provided in this book. Whether or not you have experience, get comfortable being consciously altered. How do you perceive your world when you're high? Do you think more or sense with greater awareness? I have friends who lay out questions about themselves, their wants and desires, on a pad of paper before they smoke. Then as the effects of the plant take hold, they answer the questions in the altered conscious awareness. You might find yourself surprised at some of the insights that come forth. These early steps can be your prelude to engaging the select cannabis strain you choose to explore. You will then be prepared for the encounter and open to the experience. Cannabis seems to have an innate ability to sense what we need, and with your stated intent, you've preprogrammed a cannabis-fueled event that should result in a positive outcome. Be patient and let it unfold.

In the coming months and years, you can expect plant geneticists to introduce various new strains designed specifically to enhance sexual pleasure. In fact, in those states that have recently gained legal status to grow and sell marijuana, new breeds of "sexy" strains are in development. This is excellent news for those who cannot get access to some of the strains I've listed in this book.

Take heart if you're in a state or country that hasn't legalized cannabis. Consider cannabis tourism. Plan a weekend in a city where weed is legal and discover yourself through a cannabis-infused sexual romp. When your state or country does legalize cannabis, you'll have a head start.

Sexuality is an important part of a man's health, and when properly activated it can play an important role in a variety of hormonal and synaptic processes that are important for general wellness. We feel better after sex and have greater clarity. Having multiple orgasms can open us to a new level of body awareness that until now was not a consideration. We haven't been shown how to enjoy and cultivate an awareness of our bodies and sexuality, and few if any men attend classes, read books, or watch videos on how to connect with their sensuality. As you begin to explore your sexuality through the information contained in this book, and you're able to experience a prostate orgasm, you will quickly begin to realize that you were designed to enjoy this intense pleasure as often as you like. The road map to becoming a multiorgasmic man is different for each of us. When you approach the experience with a sense of excited exploration, the rewards will come swiftly.

I wish you the best on your journey.

Resources

The items listed in this section can assist you in selecting cannabis strains and massagers and provide information to support your sexual awakening.

THE BEST WEBSITES ON CANNABIS

This short list of cannabis resources includes websites on cannabis tourism and legal issues, places to obtain strains in your area, and descriptions of different types of cannabis products.

General Information

Ashley Manta. Ashley, one of my favorite pleasure innovators, is a sex-with-cannabis advocate who developed the term *CannaSexual*. CannaSexual describes anyone who mindfully and deliberately combines sex and cannabis to enhance sensation, ease discomfort, and promote intimacy during solo or partnered play. Ashley supports men and women who are awakening to their sexual awareness and recommends topical cannabinoid-infused creams, sprays, balms, and CBD-only products.

Cannabis Life Network (CLN). This site includes resources, reviews, editorial information, a gallery, videos, and podcasts with a ton of multimedia information that is designed to keep cannabis enthusiasts informed and entertained. It covers information about marijuana throughout the world rather than just in the United States, like many of the other sites listed.

The Cannabis Chronicles. This slick and modern site, run by a grower, covers strain reviews and provides introductory cannabis information as well as information about local shops, legalization, events, and insight into the industry.

The Cannabist. This leading marijuana news website includes marijuana culture, reviews, food, and other resources. With a regular newsletter and highly active news and culture posting, it's the perfect all-in-one resource.

The Joint Blog. This blog tracks news about marijuana, ranging from new studies to legalization and focusing on issues of law and medical marijuana, including information about medical marijuana treatments, ballots, voting, and polls. It also includes guest articles and miscellaneous information that directly relate to the current marijuana industry.

Leafly. Likely the most popular marijuana site on the web, Leafly is devoted to categorizing different strains of marijuana and pointing its users to where to purchase them, if it's legal in their area. It is open to reviews and also has educational blog posts about marijuana and the industry.

My personal website, www.themaleorgasm.com, which I've packed with reviews on cannabis and massage products and articles, blogs, and galleries on a wide variety of topics featured in this book.

NORML. This is an organization that's dedicated to the reform of marijuana laws. Consequently, their site is also one of the best places to track new developments in and breaking news about marijuana legalization, such as when these issues are being voted on and the outcome of the elections. Users can also find general information about marijuana, state regulations, other legal issues, and current news releases. You can also donate, volunteer, act, and shop through the site.

Smoking with Style. This is a culturally savvy and information-heavy blog and website that includes a wide inventory of categories, such as smoking, vaping, bongs, stoner recipes, links, games, and more. It's a fun site that reviews products, gives legal information, and educates on marijuana use.

The Stoner Mom. This is one of the most unique sites on this list as it provides information about mothering and marijuana. Categories on the site include weed for beginners, podcasts, blog information, reviews, and more. It's the perfect mix of entertainment, news, and advice for mothers who enjoy either recreational or medical marijuana. It also includes some recipes for edibles and information about topics such as dabbing.

THC Finder. This site offers a marijuana blog, a finder resource, reviews, strains, and news information. Its goal is to help users find medical and recreational dispensaries, delivery services, doctors, and deals near them. It can also be used to browse the top strains that are currently popular, much like Leafly.

Toke of the Town. This is an information, entertainment, and opinion blog that includes all of the medical, cultural, dispensary, growing, and active legislation information a marijuana enthusiast needs. This website is a good all-around resource for those looking for important marijuana news and insights.

The Weed Blog. This blog compiles marijuana news and information from across the web, summarizing the events of the day and promoting an array of marijuana events. With a variety of opinion articles and other useful information, it's an all-around resource for those within the community.

Weedmaps. This is one of the better cannabis websites with details on your local dispensaries, products, and growing information.

Cannabis for Medicinal Use
Marijuana Doctors. This important blog is designed to help those who need medical marijuana. It has information about how to find a doctor, what the legalities are throughout the states, which states are pending, and resources for finding medical marijuana and getting a medical card. It covers topics such as finding a virtual marijuana doctor and dealing with federal task forces. It's the perfect resource for those who want to be aware of the laws surrounding their medicine.

Medical Marijuana Blog. This blog specifically tracks information about medical marijuana, including state laws, dispensaries, and information about benefits and growing. For medical marijuana users, this is a solid resource. It even includes a medical marijuana directory and information on how to procure a medical marijuana card.

The Cannabis Industry

420 Careers. A valuable resource, this site makes it easy to find and post listings for full- and part-time jobs within the marijuana community, and it also accepts resume submissions. It has been highly publicized, and job listings span the country and include listings for cultivators, budtenders, and marketing assistants. A blog rounds out the information that is found on this site.

Cannabis Business Blog (on the Foster Garvey website). Many companies are now going into the marijuana industry. This blog provides the information that business owners need to get into the marijuana industry safely, covering subjects ranging from legal topics around the country and taxation to regulations involving product recalls, pesticides, and the nitty-gritty of developing a business within a highly regulated industry. It also has links to a variety of other legal sites.

Growing Marijuana Blog. This blog is focused on preparations for cannabis, growing cannabis from seeds, preparing cannabis butter, and developing cannabis products. It also includes informational videos that are particularly valuable to legal medicinal users who live in states where they are allowed to grow medical marijuana in their home.

Marijuana Growing (on Jorge Cervantes site). This site provides links to thousands of resources about growing marijuana, making it very useful for new and experienced growers alike. Videos, articles, questions and answers, and an active forum make this a great resource.

Cannabis and the Law

Canna Law Group. Lawyers are getting into the business of marijuana. Though they are based in California, this group can provide legal advice for anyone interested in marijuana and the marijuana industry.

Cannabis Entertainment and Travel

Hail Mary Jane. This is a marijuana-related entertainment site. It also has a regular podcast, a directory of marijuana-related businesses, an event calendar, and a store. It is dedicated to the idea that stoners are able to be productive and happy and highlights some of the best of the community.

Pot Guide. Pot tourism is definitely a thing, and this website outlines all of the information that you need to get started. Covering Colorado, Oregon, Washington, and Nevada, it gives tourists information about where to procure pot, how to stay safe, and how to ensure that their trip is completely legal. It also has links to flight, hotel, and car rental information and maintains an active marijuana blog about general-purpose tips.

PROSTATE MASSAGERS

A Small Selection of Top Massagers

The companies listed here are some of the best massager manufacturers.

Aneros. This is the company that started it all with their patented anatomically perfect prostate massagers. The website features detailed information on how to select a massager and a men's forum for ongoing discussion on the prostate Super-O.

Doc Johnson. This line of prostate massagers includes beginning to advanced devices in an array of different sizes and shapes.

Fun Factory. Based in Germany, this manufacturer creates an excellent line of body-safe prostate toys and massagers, which are engineered for the ultimate ride.

Lovehoney. This company provides a large number of prostate massagers in all sizes and shapes.

Paloqueth. This provider makes a selection of medium-to-large prostate massagers that include a vibrating function. Ideal for noncannabis sessions, these are more expensive but for many offer a satisfying experience.

Tantus. This manufacturer was born from the aspiration to make the lives of people throughout the world fun, worthwhile, and enjoyable, and it challenges the ethos of an industry to bring what everyone truly desires—sexual happiness.

Vixen Creations. This company creates handcrafted artisan sex toys made from 100 percent platinum silicone. Products are produced in small batches and offer excellent value.

PROSTATE HEALTH

Vitamin and Mineral Supplements

Healthline. This site offers suggestions for increasing and maintaining the health of the prostate gland. The vitamins and prostate supplements listed on their site are an excellent means of staying well.

Recommended Reading

In writing this book, I've compiled the available research and data on cannabis and male sex from a wide selection of authors and research investigators. For your reading pleasure and reference, I've listed a few that might prove insightful on your journey of self-discovery.

BOOKS

Bennett, Chris. *Cannabis and the Soma Solution*. Walterville, Oregon: Trine Day, 2010.

———. *Liber 420: Cannabis, Magickal Herbs and the Occult*. Walterville, Oregon: Trine Day, 2018.

Chia, Mantak, and Douglas Abrams. *The Multi-Orgasmic Man: Sexual Secrets Every Man Should Know*. New York: HarperOne, 2009.

Chia, Mantak, and William Wei. *Chi Kung for Prostate Health and Sexual Vigor*. Rochester, Vt.: Destiny Books, 2013.

Glickman, Charlie, and Aislinn Emirzian. *The Ultimate Guide to Prostate Pleasure*. Berkeley: Cleis Press, 2013.

Gray, Steven. *Cannabis and Spirituality*. Rochester, Vt.: Inner Traditions, 2017.

Holland, Julie. *The Pot Book: A Complete Guide to Cannabis*. Rochester, Vt.: Park Street Press, 2018.

Johnson, Will. *Cannabis in Spiritual Practice*. Rochester, Vt.: Inner Traditions, 2018.

Lewis, Barbara. *The Sexual Powers of Marijuana*. New York: Wyden, 1973.

Wilson, Robert Anton. *Sex & Drugs: A Journey Beyond Limits*. Sedona, Ariz.: New Falcon Publications, 1973.

ARTICLES

Alger, Bradley. "Getting High on the Endocannabinoid System." *Cerebrum* (December 2013): 14.

Aneros Wiki. June 11, 2021.

Awaken Consciousness website. "How the Brain and Orgasm Conspire in Consciousness." June 13, 2016.

Bazar, Ronald. "10 Amazing Functions of the Prostate Gland." Prostate.net website. February 17, 2012.

The Big Gay Review website. "Prostate Massage: A Buyers Guide." September 22, 2014.

Ella Paradis website. "How to Have a Prostate Orgasm: Our Guide to Prostate Milking." May 30, 2018.

Engle, Gigi. "10 Men Reveal What It's Like to Get Off with a Prostate Massager." February 28, 2019. Men's Health website.

Like a Porn Star website. "How to Choose a Prostate Massager." October 8, 2019.

Little, Callie. "How Weed Can Supercharge Your Sex Life." Thrillist website. December 1, 2016.

Mandelbaum, Ryan. "Man Had So Many Prostate Orgasms He Couldn't Stop, According to a New Paper." Gizmodo website. December 21, 2017.

Manta, Ashley. "Can Cannabis Give You Multiple Orgasms?" Leafly website. May 7, 2016.

———. "Cannabis and Mind Blowing Sex." Ashley Manta website. November 18, 2015.

Monteiro, Amanda. "Neuroscientist: Orgasms Can Be Used to Reach an Altered State of Consciousness." Collective Evolution website. September 26, 2017.

Necco, Terry. "Marijuana and Sex: A Classic Combination." Cannabis Culture website. September 1, 1998.

PinkCherry. "Prostate Massager Guide for Beginners." PinkCherry website. December 24, 2019.

PlantedU website. "Cannabis Terpenes: What They Are and How They Work." June 21, 2018.

Index